Generis

PUBLISHING

I0110146

Cervical Cancer:
Awareness, knowledge, and vaccination hesitancy

The main author: Tassang Andrew

Co-authors: Halle-Ekane GE, Nembulefack D, Ewane T, Tassang T, Ewang Ebong C, Enow- Orock A E, Folefac L, Ndaka W, Ncham G, Cho Fred, Ngum Fru P

Title: Cervical Cancer: Awareness, knowledge, and vaccination hesitancy

ISBN: 978-1-63902-652-4

Author: Tassang Andrew

Cover image: www.pixabay.com

Generis Publishing
Online orders: www.generis-publishing.com
Orders by email: info@generis-publishing.com

TABLE OF CONTENTS

CHAPTER I

CERVICAL CANCER SCREENING IN A LOW – RESSOURCE SETTING: BUEA- CAMEROON

Tassang A, Halle-Ekane GE, Nembulefack D, Ewane T, Tassang T, Ewang Ebong C, Enow- Orock A E, Folefac L, Ndaka W, Ncham G, Cho Fred, Ngum Fru P

ACKNOWLEDGEMENT

We would like to express our heartfelt gratitude to the Cameroon Arizona Partnership program and most specially to Associate Professor Mike Brady and Dr. David Greenspan of Arizona University for their physical, material and technical support. Without their care and funding, it would have been so difficult to accomplish this task.

Our regards of appreciation also go to the all the staffs of Buea regional hospital who were involved in the preparation and execution of this screening campaign. Many thanks to its director.

ABSTRACT

Introduction: Cervical cancer is the second most common gynecological cancer in low-income countries. Its burden is still huge in Cameroon, largely due to the absence of a nationwide prevention program. Visual inspection of the cervix with acetic acid and Lugol's iodine is an acceptable, effective, and affordable screening method in low-income countries. We aim at increasing the uptake of cervical cancer screening in the Buea Health Area, by establishing an operational cervical cancer clinic at the Buea Regional Hospital.

Methods: We conducted a single day cervical cancer screening and treatment clinic at the Buea Regional Hospital on the 2nd November, 2019. Thermal coagulation and LEEP were available treatment options for dysplastic lesions. A MobileODT colposcopic device was used to enhanced visualization of the cervix. Data was entered into Microsoft Excel 2016 and exported to Epi Info version 7 for statistical analysis.

Results: A total of 140 women opted to participate in the study. Amongst them, 124 completed the screening procedure giving a screening uptake of 88.6%. Of those screened, the mean age was 36.53(±12.17), and majority (97.6%) reported negative for HIV. Eight (6.5%) participants screened positive, LSIL 7(5.6%) and HSIL 1(0.8%).

Although 111 (89.5%) participants believed that cervical cancer is preventable, only 37 (29.8%) had been previously screened and just one had previously been vaccinated against HPV. Two positive cases met treatment eligibility criteria, however, only one accepted treatment given a treatment uptake of 50%. The HSIL lesion was treated by excision and histopathology result later confirmed CIN 2.

Conclusion: With increasing awareness that cervical cancer is a preventable disease, uptake of vaccination, screening, and treatment measures are still very low. Single day screening and treatment clinic will improve on cervical cancer screening uptake in most low-income countries, prior to the implementation of effective nationwide screening programs.

Keywords: Cervical Cancer, single day screening and treatment, Visual Inspection with Acetic acid and Lugol's iodine, Thermal coagulation, LEEP, Buea.

INTRODUCTION

Cervical cancer is a global health burden, ranked as the second most common and deadliest gynecological cancer in low-income countries [1]. The global incidence of cervical cancer is approximately 529,409 new cases, and more than half of these new cases die annually [1]. In Cameroon, more than 6 million sexually active women are at risk of developing cervical cancer, there are 1993 newly diagnosed cases annually, and over 55% of these cases die annually despite the fact that cervical cancer is a preventable disease [2].

Cervical dysplasia or pre-cancer lesions are the abnormal precursor cells which can later progress to frank cervical cancer [3]. The peak incidence of cervical dysplasia occurs within the ages of 25 to 35 years [4]. If diagnosed early, most of these dysplastic cells can be treated successfully, hence preventing further progression to invasive cervical cancer [5]. The Human Papilloma Virus (HPV) is regarded as the main causative agent of cervical pre-cancer lesions [5]. Despite the presence of a vaccine against HPV, its availability and affordability is still very low in Cameroon and most other low-income countries [6].

The American College of Obstetricians and Gynecologist recommend first screening for cervical dysplasia to begin at age 21 years, regardless of age at sexual initiation or other behavioral risk factors [7]. However, fewer than 19% of women have been screened in low-income countries [8]. In Cameroon, cervical cancer screening is not routinely carried-out in most healthcare services, and no nationwide screening program have been implemented by the government. In 2007, the Cameroon Baptist Convention Health Services launched the Women Health Program which have ever since champion the screening of cervical cancer in most region of the country using the visual inspection technique, and enhance by digital cervicography [9]. Beside insufficient screening programs, the cost of screening, the lack of information on screening programs, the notion that the screening process is painful, have been reported as some of the factors responsible for the low uptake of cervical cancer screening in Cameroon [10].

Visual inspection of the cervix with acetic acid (VIA) has been reported as an effective, and affordable screening test that can be combined with simple treatment methods for early cervical lesions eradication [11]. There is the need for the utilization of such screening method, as screening a woman just once with VIA between the ages of 30 and 49 years have been reported to decrease her lifetime risk of developing invasive cervical cancer by 26% [12]. Also, increasing cervical cancer screening through visual inspection with acetic acid and Lugol's iodine (VIA/VILI) with trained personnel may increase the uptake and coverage of cervical cancer screening [13]. As a measure to increase the uptake of cervical cancer screening in the Buea health area, we organized a free cervical cancer screening campaign at the Buea Regional Hospital using the VIA/VILLI technique, and with the help of a MobileODT colposcopic device to enhance the visualization of positive lesions [14]. This screening campaign is one of a series of projects required to fully established a functional cervical cancer clinic at the Buea Regional Hospital, and subsequently to other parts of the South West Region of Cameroon. This program is an initiative of the Buea Regional Hospital and the Cameroon-Arizona Partnership, with a common vision of decreasing maternal mortality via early screening and treatment of cervical dysplastic lesions by trained local healthcare personnel.

METHOD

Study Design and Setting

This was a single day screen-and-treat cervical cancer clinic carried-out on the 2nd November 2019 at the Buea Regional Hospital in the South West Region of Cameroon.

The Buea Regional Hospital is a 120 bed capacity intermediate level referral hospital located in Buea, at the foot of Mount Cameroon. It is a government-own hospital, which serves as a clinical rotation site for the University of Buea Medical School. It is the lone referral hospital for the Buea health area which has an estimated population of over 200 000 inhabitants [15]. Under the patronage of the University of Buea in partnership with the University of Arizona School of Medicine Phoenix, a "Cancer Screening and Early Diagnostic Center" is being created at the Buea Regional Hospital. This site is run by a handful healthcare workers and overseen by a pathologist and a couple of gynecologists with ASCCP certification. This health unit was used as the screening site during this cervical cancer screening clinic. Administrative approval to carry-out this screening campaign was obtained from the South West Regional Delegation of Public Health.

Study Population and Procedure

All women who were at least 21 years of age were invited for this screening via radio announcements, public banners and social media campaigns. Our exclusion criteria were, pregnancy, history of prior total hysterectomy and women aged above 65 years. Upon arrival, potential participants were informed about the screening procedure before they were allowed to sign a consent form and enroll for the screening. They were also assured that they had the right to withdraw their consent at any stage of the screening process. Prior to the screening proper, a data collection sheet was used to collect information on demography, gyno-obstetrical history, awareness and previous exposure to the risk factors of cervical cancer. We had 3 screening stations, two were run by obstetrician/gynecologists, and the third station was run by a trained general practitioner. An ASCCP trained colposcopist supervised these screening stations. The women lied in a lithotomy position on an examination bed, and the external genitalia was examined before placing a sterile plastic speculum into the vaginal to enable a clear visualization of the cervix and the transformation zone. A freshly prepared 5% acetic acid was applied on the cervix, and after 1 minute it was observed with the naked eyes and with the MobileODT colposcopic device. Findings were described as negative or positive based on the WHO/IARC practical manual on visual screening for cervical neoplasia [16]. Preliminary photos were taken for all VIA positive cases before application of Lugol's iodine. All VIA positive cases were confirmed positive with VILI before treatment was initiated. Results were reported as negative, low-grade squamous intraepithelial lesion (LSIL), high grade squamous intraepithelial lesion (HSIL), and suspicious for cancer. All patients with HSIL were treated with Loop Electrical Excision Procedure (LEEP), and samples sent for histopathology. All participants ≥ 25 years of age with a LSIL were eligible for thermal coagulation in accordance with the current WHO eligibility guidelines [17]. Participants with LSIL who were below 25 years old did not benefit from any treatment option, but were to be re-evaluated in one year according to the WHO/IARC beginners manual [18]. All negative cases were offered a 3-year rendezvous for rescreening. Biopsy was to be provided to all cases with suspicion of cancer. At the end of the screening process, participants were all provided with their screening result, instructions on subsequent follow-up, and when next to go for screening.

Data entry and analysis

Data was entered into a Microsoft Excel spreadsheet and exported to Epi Info version 7 for analysis. Categorical variables were expressed as frequencies and percentages. Continuous variables were expressed as mean and standard deviation. Two-tailed Fisher exact test was used to determine association between screening results and participants' characteristics. A p-value < 0.05 was considered to be statistically significant.

RESULTS

Participants' Characteristics

One hundred and forty (140) women opted to participate in this screening program. However, 16 women withdrew their consent in the course of the process, and declined from undergoing the screening procedure. A total of 124 participants completed the screening procedure, given a screening uptake of 88.6%. Among those who initially opted to participate in the screening, the mean age was 35.81 (±12.37); forty-eight (34.3%) of them were married, and 91 (65.0%) had attained university level of education.

Among those who completed the screening, the mean age was 36.53 (±12.17), with up to 50 (40.3%) of them in the 21- 30 years' age group. Forty-five (36.3%) were married, and 79 (63.7%) had attained university level of education. The majority, 121 (97.6%) of these participants reported a negative HIV serology result. Although 37 (29.8%) of these participants had previously been screened for cervical cancer, only 1 (0.8%) of them admitted to have been vaccinated against HPV. Among those who had been screened before, only one person reported a prior positive result, and the lesion was treated by excision.

Table 1 summarizes the characteristics of participants who completed the screening procedure.

Table 1. Characteristics of participants who completed the screening (N=124)

Variables	Responses	Frequency, (n)	Percentages, (%)
Age group	21-30	50	40.3
	31-40	25	20.2
	41-50	29	23.4
	51-60	17	13.7
	61-65	3	2.4
Marital status	Married	45	36.3
	Single	72	58.1
	Divorced	3	2.4
	Widow	4	3.2
Educational level	Primary	14	11.3
	Secondary	31	25.0
	University	79	63.7
Parity	Multipara	46	37.1
	Nulliparara/Primipara	78	62.9
Age of first intercourse	<21 years	83	76.2
	>21 years	26	23.9
Multiple sexual partners in the last 5 years	Yes	61	49.2
	No	63	50.8
History of genital warts	Yes	25	20.2
	No	99	79.8
Reported HIV status	Negative	121	97.6
	Positive	3	2.4
Use of contraceptives	Yes	9	7.3
	No	115	92.7
Previous screening for cervical cancer	Yes	37	29.8
	No	87	70.2
Previously vaccinated for HPV	Yes	1	0.8
	No	123	99.2

Screening results and treatment modalities

As shown in Figure 1, eight (6.5%) participants screened positive for cervical squamous intraepithelial lesion. Seven (5.6%) of those screened positive had low-grade lesion and only 1 (0.8%) case was diagnosed as high-grade lesion. Of those with low-grade lesion, 6 were within 21 to 24 years of age. Of the 8 participants who screened positive, 2 were eligible for treatment. The first was a 38 years old with LSIL who met eligibility criteria for thermal coagulation, and the second was the lone HSIL case at 40 years of age who met eligibility criteria for LEEP. The case of HSIL underwent LEEP and sample was sent for histopathology which confirmed CIN 2. However, the LSIL case who was eligible for thermal coagulation did not consent for treatment. The only participant who previously screened positive and benefitted from excision therapy had a negative test result during this screening program. All cases screened positive were to be reviewed in 1 year.

Table 2 displays participants results according to age group.

Table 2. Screening results of participants

Age group, (Years)	VIA/VILI Results (N=124)			
	Negative (n=116)	Positive (n=8)		Total
		LSIL	HSIL	Frequency, (%)
21-30	44	6	0	50 (40.3)
31-40	23	1	1	25 (20.2)
41-50	29	0	0	29 (23.4)
51-60	17	0	0	17 (13.7)
61-65	3	0	0	3 (2.4)

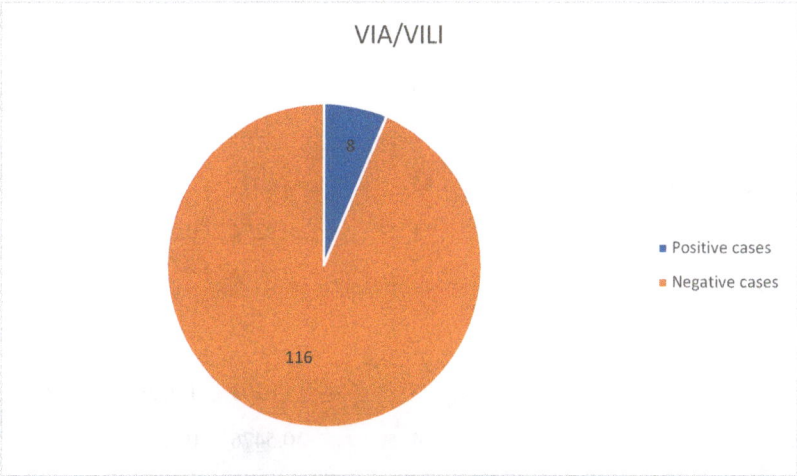

Figure 1. Graphical display of the proportion of positive and negative cases.

Screening and Prevention Beliefs

Among those screened, 111 (89.5%) believed that cervical cancer is a preventable disease. The majority 101 (81.5%) also believed that infection with HPV increases one's lifetime chance of developing cervical cancer. Also, 82 (66.1%) of these participants believed that there is a vaccine against HPV, which serve as the primary preventive method for cervical cancer.

Relationship between participants' characteristics and screening results

As shown in Table 3, bivariate analysis was used to assess the association between a positive screening result and participants' characteristic. Participants with age ≤ 35 years had the highest odds of being screened positive, with 3 times more risk than those above 35 years. However, this correlation was not statistically significant (P-value = 0.15). Higher odds of being screened positive was also reported for those with multiple sexual partners in the last 5 years, and those who had only attained primary or secondary level of education. Also, participants with a history of screening had a lesser chance of being screened positive (OR= 0.7714). Parity, history of genital warts, age of first intercourse < 21 years were not positively associated with a positive screening result in this study.

Table 3. Correlation between participants' characteristics and results of screening (N=124)

Characteristics		VIA/VILI Positive	VIA/VILI Negative	Odds Ratio	Relative Risk	P-value
Age	≤ 35 years	6	53	3.5660	3.3051	0.15
	≥ 36 years	2	63			
Age of first intercourse	< 21 years	4	79	0.4684	0.4940	0.44
	≥ 21 years	4	37			
Parity	Multipara	1	45			
	Nullipara/ primipara	7	71	0.2254	0.2422	0.26
Level of education	Primary/ secondary	4	41			
	University	4	75	1.8293	1.7556	0.46
History of genital warts	Yes	1	24	0.5476	0.5657	1.00
	No	7	92			
Multiple sexual partners < 5 years.	Yes	5	56	1.7857	1.7213	0.49
	No	3	60			
History of screening	Yes	2	35	0.7714	0.7838	1.00
		6	81			

DISCUSSION

The mean age of those screened was 36.53 years. Similar mean age among participants was also reported by Horo et al. in Ivory Coast [19]. However, Tebeu et al. reported a higher mean age of 41.59 years in a study carried-out in six regions in Cameroon [20]. This difference could be due to the fact that they included only women who were at least 25 years of age. We had a screening uptake of 88.6% in this study; similar level of screening uptake as also reported by Horo et al. in Ivory Coast [19].

The prevalence of abnormal cervical lesion (dysplasia) was 6.5% in this study, and majority of the positive cases were LSIL (5.6%). Eakin et al. reported a prevalence of 6.09%, with LSIL being 5.2% [21]. These similarities could be due to the fact that these two studies were done in the same town. However, Abdul et al in Nigeria, and Kafuruki et al. in Tanzania reported a prevalence of abnormal cervical lesion of 14% and 26.8% respectively [22,1]. This higher prevalence could be due to the fact that, these studies were carried-out among chronic pelvic inflammatory disease and HIV patients respectively. In this study, one out of two showed up for treatment which was lower than the uptake of 100% obtained by Eakin et al. [21] This discrepancy could result from the fact that almost all of their participants had attained university level of education, hence has a better understanding of the need for treatment if found positive.

Almost 90% of our participants' belief that cervical cancer is a preventable disease, but only 29.8% had been screened for cervical cancer. Similar patterns of low screening uptake despite increased awareness that cervical cancer is a preventable disease was reported in other low-income countries [23]. Over 65% of these participants' belief that there is a vaccine against HPV, but just one person had been vaccinated. Very low rate of vaccination against HPV was also reported in neighboring Nigeria [24]. This could be due to the unavailability and in affordability of this vaccine among this population. There is therefore the need for free vaccination campaigns, and prevention programs in order to increase uptake of HPV vaccines.

With regards to participants' characteristic which could predispose them to a positive result, age <35 years had a higher probability of being screened positive though this was not statistically significant. This confirms with current literature which states that the peak incidence of cervical dysplasia is within 25 to 35 years. This was however contrary to findings by Tebeu et al., and Avidime et al. who reported a higher incidence of dysplasia among those with age > 30 years [20,25]. Also, participants who had only attained primary or secondary level of education had a higher chance of being screened positive, though this difference was not statistically significant. DeGregorio et al. also reported that participants with a low educational status had a higher probability of being screened positive of precancerous lesions [9]. This aligns with previous

15

literature, stating that low educational status increases vulnerability to poor sexual practices and consequently increase exposure to HPV infection. Having multiple sexual partners within the last 5 years was also found to increases the possibility of being screened positive. Similar findings were also reported in another study in East Africa [1].

More so, age of initiation of coitus < 21 years was not positively related to being screen positive for precancerous lesion in this study. Similar findings were reported by Abdul et al. in 2009 in Nigeria [22]. On the contrary, DeGregorio et al. found out that, early age of sexual debut was associated with positive VIA results [9]. This discrepancy could be due to the fact that, they carried-out a retrospective study involving over forty-six thousand participants. Lastly, participants with a previous history of screening showed lesser chances of being screened VIA/VILI positive during subsequent screenings, hence, re-enforcing on the need for regular cervical cancer screenings in accordance with standard guidelines.

CONCLUSION

The prevalence of cervical dysplastic lesions in this study was 6.5%. Most of those who screened positive were less than 35 years of age. Uptake of vaccination, screening, and treatment practices are still low despite increased awareness that cervical cancer is preventable.

 Participants with multiple sexual partners, and those with low level of education were more likely to be screened positive for dysplasia.

Single day screening and treatment clinic could serve as an important step in improving cervical cancer screening and enhance prevention in most low-income countries, prior to the implementation of effective nationwide screening program.

REFERENCES

1. Kafuruki L, Rambau PF, Massinde A, Masalu N. Prevalence and predictors of Cervical Intraepithelial Neoplasia among HIV infected women at Bugando Medical Centre, Mwanza-Tanzania. Infect Agent Cancer. 2013;8:45.
2. Cameroon: Human Papillomavirus and Related Diseases, Summary Report 2015 - CMR.pdf. [cited 2020 Feb 10]. Available from: http://www.hpvcentre.net/statistics/reports/CMR.pdf

3. Enow-Orock G, Mbu R, Ngowe NM, Tabung FK, Mboudou E, Ndom P, et al. Gynecological cancer profile in the Yaounde population, Cameroon. Clin Mother Child Health. 2006;3(1):437–44.

4. Dunn TS, Bajaj JE, Stamm CA, Beaty B. Management of the Minimally Abnormal Papanicolaou Smear in Pregnancy. J Low Genit Tract Dis. 2001;5(3):133–7.

5. Cervical dysplasia. University of Maryland Medical Center. 2015. Available from: https://umm.edu/health/medical/altmed/condition/cervical-dysplasia

6. Ogembo J, Manga S, Nulah K, Foglabenchi L, Perlman S, Wamai R, et al. Achieving high uptake of human papillomavirus vaccine in Cameroon: Lessons learned in overcoming challenges - ScienceDirect. [cited 2020 Feb 14]. Available from: https://www.sciencedirect.com/science/article/pii/S0264410X14008652

7. Randel A. ACOG Releases Guidelines on Cervical Cancer Screening. Am Fam Physician. 2013;88(11):776–7.

8. Gakidou E, Nordhagen S, Obermeyer Z. Coverage of Cervical Cancer Screening in 57 Countries: Low Average Levels and Large Inequalities. PLOS Med. 2008;5(6):e132.

9. DeGregorio GA, Bradford LS, Manga S, Tih PM, Wamai R, Ogembo R, et al. Prevalence, Predictors, and Same Day Treatment of Positive VIA Enhanced by Digital Cervicography and Histopathology Results in a Cervical Cancer Prevention Program in Cameroon. PLOS ONE. 2016;11(6):e0157319.

10. Halle-Ekane GE, Nembulefack DK, Orock GE, Fon PN, Tazinya AA, Tebeu PM. Knowledge of Cervical Cancer and Its Risk Factors, Attitudes and Practices towards Pap Smear Screening among Students in the University of Buea, Cameroon. J Cancer Tumor Int. 2018;1–11.

11. ACCP_screening_factsheet_2009.pdf. [cited 2020 Feb 16]. Available from: https://www.paho.org/hq/dmdocuments/2011/ACCP_screening_factsheet_2009.pdf

12. Goldie SJ, Kuhn L, Denny L, Pollack A, Wright TC. Policy Analysis of Cervical Cancer Screening Strategies in Low-Resource Settings: Clinical Benefits and Cost-effectiveness. JAMA. 2001;285(24):3107–15.

13. Poli UR, Bidinger PD, Gowrishankar S. Visual Inspection with Acetic Acid (VIA) Screening Program: 7 Years Experience in Early Detection of Cervical Cancer and Pre-Cancers in Rural South India. Indian J Community Med Off Publ Indian Assoc Prev Soc Med. 2015;40(3):203–7.

14. MobileODT | The Smart Mobile Colposcope. MobileODT. [cited 2020 Feb 16]. Available from: https://www.mobileodt.com

15. BUEA. [cited 2020 Feb 16]. Available from: http://cvuc.cm/national/index.php/en/about-uccc/the-secretariat/142-association/carte-administrative/sud-ouest/fako/404-buea

16. Sankaranarayanan R, Wesley RS, International Agency for Research on Cancer. A practical manual on visual screening for cervical neoplasia. Lyon: International Agency for Research on Cancer, World Health Organization; 2003.

17. WHO | Comprehensive cervical cancer control. WHO. [cited 2020 Feb 14]. Available from: http://www.who.int/reproductivehealth/publications/cancers/cervical-cancer-guide/en/

18. Colposcopy and treatment of cervical intraepithelial neoplasia: a beginners' manual. [cited 2020 Feb 16]. Available from: https://screening.iarc.fr/colpochap.php?lang=1&chap=11.php

19. Horo AG, Didi-Kouko Coulibaly J, Koffi A, Tchounga B, Seni K, Aka KE, et al. Cervical Cancer Screening Program by Visual Inspection: Acceptability and Feasibility in Health Insurance Companies. Obstet Gynecol Int. 2015;2015:1–4.

20. Tebeu P, Sando Z, Ndoumba A, Sandjong I, Mawech-Fauceglia P, Doh AS. Prevalence and Geographical Distribution of Precancerous Lesions of the Uterine Cervix in Cameroon. J Cytol Histol. 2013 [cited 2020 Feb 16];2013. Available from: http://www.omicsonline.org/cytology-histology-abstract.php?abstract_id=19109

21. Eakin C, Ekollo R, Nembulefack D, Halle-Ekane G, Tangui G, Brady R, et al. Cervical Cancer Screening Beliefs and Prevalence of LSIL/HSIL Among a University-Based Population in Cameroon. J Low Genit Tract Dis. 2018;22(4):274–279.

22. Abdul MA, Shittu SO, Randawa JA, Shehu MS. The cervical smear pattern in patients with chronic pelvic inflammatory disease. Niger J Clin Pract. 2009;12(3):289–93.

23. Pengpid S, Peltzer K. Attitudes and Practice of Cervical Cancer Screening among Female University Students from 25 Low, Middle Income and Emerging Economy Countries. Asian Pac J Cancer Prev APJCP. 2014;15:7235–9.

24. Wright KO, Aiyedehin O, Akinyinka MR, Ilozumba O. Cervical Cancer: Community Perception and Preventive Practices in an Urban Neighborhood of Lagos (Nigeria). Int Sch Res Not. 2014;2014:e950534.

25. Avidime S, Ahmed S, Oguntayo A, Abu T, Ndako J. Pattern of cervical dysplasia among women of reproductive age in Zaria, Northern Nigeria. ResearchGate. 2014 [cited 2020 Feb 20]. Available from: https://www.researchgate.net/publication/265085786_Pattern_of_cervical_dyspl asia_among_women_of_reproductive_age_in_Zaria_Northern_Nigeria

CHAPTER II

SOCIO-ECONOMIC DETERMINANTS INFLUENCING CERVICAL CANCER SCREENING IN BUEA:

A CROSS-SECTIONAL STUDY

Neh Fru C, Tassang A, Cho F, Tassang T, Ngum Fru P

ABSTRACT

Introduction

Cervical cancer remains a huge burden in scarce resource communities as ours. The morbidity and mortality are enormous, despite the preventable nature of this pathology.

This study set to explore the socioeconomic variables which could help influence positively presentation for screening, which will in turn lessen the pressure on our fragile heath system.

Methodology

A one-day free screening campaign was organized at the Buea regional hospital. After thorough explanation of the exercise to the potential participants to this study, a questionnaire was distributed to them. Assurance was given about the confidentiality of this study, and they were also informed that, they could opt out at any moment, if they so wish.

Results

Some of the socioeconomic variables influencing presentation for cervical cancer screening were identified. They were namely: age, level of education, residence, marital status, age at first sexual intercourse, number of sexual partners, number of pregnancies and number of deliveries.

Conclusion

Understanding and acting on these variables could help curb down morbidity and mortality, thus alleviating the burden on our fragile heath system.

Key words: cancer of the cervix, socioeconomic variables, influencing participation, screening.

INTRODUCTION

Cancer of the cervix is fast becoming a very heavy burden both clinically and financially in the developing countries (1). It is the 2nd gynecological cancer in women worldwide and is responsible for heavy morbidity and mortality (2).

There are about 528.000 cases of cervical cancer occurring all over the world with 266.000 deaths annually. 85% of these cases occur in the developing world. (3).

This disease is essentially preventable, given its natural course. The Bethesda classification of cervical cancer ranges from normal cervix, derangement of cells of no specified significance, Low Grade Lesion, High Grade lesion then finally Infiltrating Cancer (3). The evolution from one stage to the next, is very gradual, and may take up to 10 years (4, 5).

Cervical cancer can be preventable by primary measures which are screening, and vaccination. The secondary measure is detection of an early abnormality through screening and treatment of the pre-invasive lesions. (6)

In Cameroon about 6.00.000 women are sexually active, and are at risk of developing cancer of the cervix. 1993 new cases are diagnosed per year, and over 55% of these cases die annually, despite the fact that cancer of the cervix is highly preventable. (7).

Given the fact that cancer of the cervix is not a disease of sudden unset, we were interested in this study, to find out, what socioeconomically could influence members the community to present themselves for a cervical cancer screening exercise as a preventive measure.

Are there socio-economic factors which are responsible for the low turn out for cervical cancer screening?

A free campaign for cervical cancer screening was organized in Buea regional hospital, this study took into consideration among others the following socioeconomic variables; age, level of education, marital status, occupation, residence, number of sexual partners for the last 5 years, age of first intercourse., number of deliveries and pregnancies.

METHODOLOGY

Study Design and Setting

Buea is the capital city of the South West region of Cameroon, built at the foot of Mount Cameroon which stands majestically at 4100 m above the sea level. This town harbours one of the regional hospitals of the region. This health institution is of intermediate level, and serves as a teaching hospital for students of the Faculty of Health of the state university bearing same name as the town. It is the lone referral hospital for the Buea health area with a population of 200.000 inhabitants (8).

The Buea regional hospital, alongside the Cameroon Arizona partnership program; a collaborative platform between the university of Buea and the University of Arizona School of Medicine Phoenix, organized a single day of "see and treat" free cervical cancer screening campaign on the 2nd of November 2019.

Ethical and administrative approval

The ethical clearance was given by the department of obstetrics and gynecology of the university of Buea.

Next, the dean of the faculty of health requested and obtained an administrative clearance from the regional delegation of public health Buea.

Study Population and Procedure

Women aged at least 21 years of age were invited for this screening exercise via radio announcements, public banners and social media campaigns. Exclusion criteria for this study were, pregnancy, history of prior hysterectomy and women aged above 66 years. Upon arrival, potential participants were informed about the screening procedure before they were allowed to sign a consent form and enroll for the screening. All participants in this study were informed in details about the objective of this study and time involvement. Any participant had the right to leave the study at any time. A written consent was obtained from all the participants. Anonymity and privacy was ensured while collecting data for this study. Care was taken not to cause any harm or discomfort to all the respondents.

A data collection sheet was used to collect information on demography, education, socioeconomic background, gynea-obstetrical history, and previous exposure to the risk factors of cervical cancer.

Statistical analysis

We entered data into and analysed with IBM-SPSS Statistics 21.0 for windows (IBM-SPSS Corp., Chicago USA). The Chi square (χ^2) test was used to compare socio-demographic characteristics with previous cervical cancer screening and stepwise multinomial logistic regression to identify significant correlates of the main sociodemographic covariates. Only covariates with χ^2 p-values of 0.21 were included in the multinomial regression analysis. p-values ≤ 0.05 were considered significant.

RESULTS

CHARTS AND TABLES

Table 1: Socio-demographic characteristics of study participants

Variable	Subclass	Frequency (%)
Age groups (Years)	≤ 30 (16 – 30)	61 (43.6)
	31 – 40	26 (18.6)
	41 – 50	32 (22.9)
	> 50 (51 – 66)	21 (15.0)
	Total	140
Education	Primary	14 (10.1)
	Secondary	34 (24.6)
	Tertiary	90 (65.2)
	Total	138
Occupation	Skilled	64 (46.0)
	Business	12 (8.6)
	Unskilled/ Unemployed	15 (10.8)
	Student	48 (34.5)
	Total	139
Marital status	Unmarried	89 (65.0)
	Married	48 (35.0)
	Total	137
Locality	Rural	29 (20.9)
	Semi urban	33 (23.7)
	Urban	77 (55.4)
	Total	139

Table 2: Association of number of pregnancies/ deliveries with previous screening

		Previous screening			
G	Yes (%)	No (%)	Total (%)	$\chi 2$	p - value
0 – 4 pregnancies	25 (71.4)	83 (86.5)	108 (82.4)	4.003	0.045*
5 –10 pregnancies	10 (28.6)	13 (13.5)	108 (82.4)		
Total	35	96	131		
P					
0 – 3 deliveries	26 (74.3)	86 (89.6)	112 (85.5)	4.840	0.028*
4 – 8 deliveries	9 (25.7)	10 (10.4)	19 (14.5)		
Total	35	96	131		
Age of first sex					
< 20 years	21 (61.8)	49 (57.0)	70 (58.3)	0.334	0.6 (0.2 – 1.7)
≥ 20 years	13 (38.2)	37 (43.0)	50 (41.7)	Ref	1.0
Total	34	86	120		
Number of sex partners					
> 1 partner	8 (22.2)	48 (54.5)	56 (45.2)	0.027*	4.9 (1.2 – 20.7)
0 – 1 partner	28 (77.8)	40 (45.5)	68 (54.8)	Ref	1.0
Total	36	88	124		

Table 3: Determinants to cervical cancer screening

VARIABLE	DV: Previously screened for cervical cancer				
Age groups (Years)	**Yes (%)**	**No (%)**	**Total (%)**	***p*-value**	**O.R (95% C.I)**
≤ 30 (16 – 30)	5 (13.2)	56 (55.4)	61 (43.9)	0.050*	7.9 (1.0 – 63.5)†
31 – 40	6 (15.8)	20 (19.8)	26 (18.7)	0.031*	7.8 (1.2 – 50.4)†
41 – 50	15 (39.5)	16 (15.8)	31 (22.3)	0.25	2.5 (0.5 – 12.4)†
> 50 (51 – 66)	12 (31.6)	9 (8.9)	21 (15.1)	Ref	1.0
Total	38	101	139		

Education	6 (15.8)	8 (8.1)	14 (10.2)	0.261	3.2 (0.4 – 24.7) †
Primary	13 (34.2)	21 (21.2)	34 (24.8)	0.047*	0.3 (0.1 – 1.0)
Secondary	19 (50.0)	70 (70.7)	89 (65.0)	Ref	1.0
Tertiary	19 (50.0)	70 (70.7)	89 (65.0)		
Total	38	99	137		
Locality					
Rural	7 (18.4)	22 (21.8)	29 (20.9)	0.886	1.1 (0.3 – 4.5)
Semi urban	10 (26.3)	23 (22.8)	33 (23.7)	0.419	1.6 (0.5 – 5.6) †
Urban	21 (55.3)	56 (55.4)	77 (55.4)	Ref	1.0
Total	38	101	139		
Occupation					
Skilled	24 (63.2)	39 (39.0)	63 (45.7)	0.601	0.6 (0.1 – 4.2)
Business	6 (15.8)	6 (6.0)	12 (8.7)	0.114	0.1 (0.0 – 1.6)
Unskilled/ Unemployed	5 (13.2)	10 (10.0)	15 (10.9)	0.966	1.0 (0.1 – 11.3) †
Student	3 (7.9)	45 (45.0)	48 (34.8)	Ref	1.0
Total	38	100	138		
Marital status					
Unmarried	19 (51.4)	70 (70.7)	89 (65.4)	0.526	0.7 (0.2 – 2.2)
Married	18 (48.6)	29 (28.9)	47 (34.6)	Ref	1.0
Total	37	99	136		
Age of first sex					
< 20 years	21 (61.8)	49 (57.0)	70 (58.3)	0.334	0.6 (0.2 – 1.7)
≥ 20 years	13 (38.2)	49 (57.0)	50 (41.7)	Ref	1.0
Total	34	86	120		
Number of sex partners					
> 1 partner	8 (22.2)	48 (54.5)	56 (45.2)	0.027*	4.9 (1.2 – 20.7)
0 – 1 partner	28 (77.8)	40 (45.5)	68 (54.8)	Ref	1.0
Total	36	88	124		

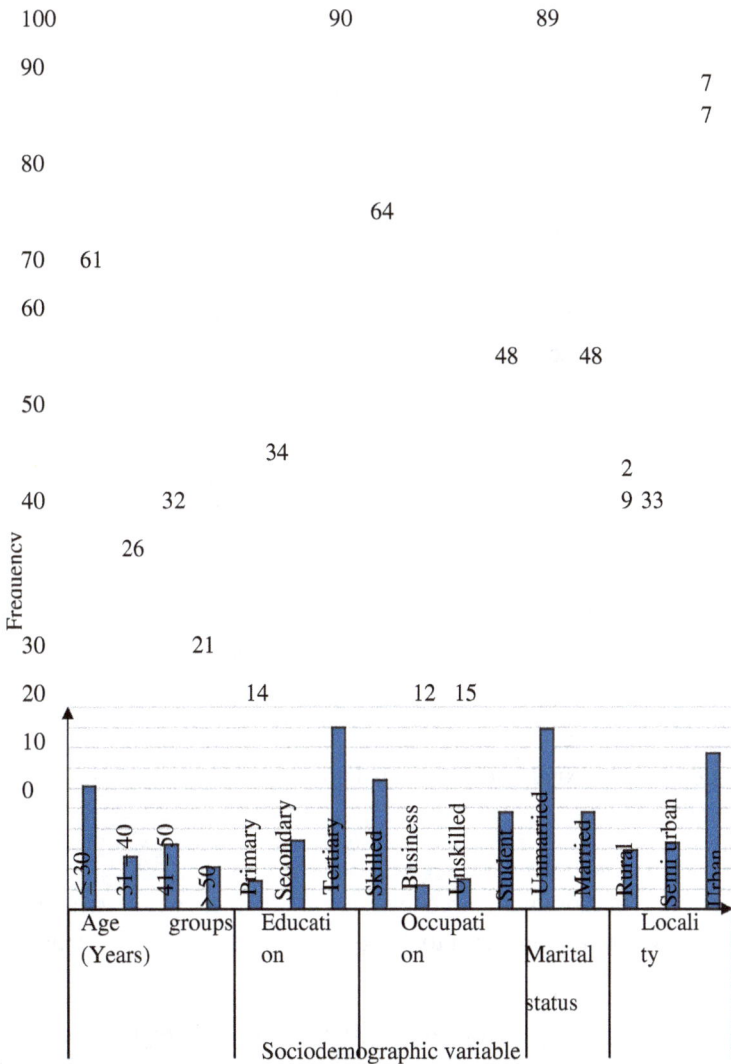

100				90		89	
90							7
							7
80						
				64		
70	61					
60						48	48
50						
			34				2
40		32				9	33
	26					
30		21				
20			14		12	15
10						
0						

Frequency

Age (Years) groups — <30, 31 – 40, 41 – 50, >50

Education — Primary, Secondary, Tertiary

Occupation — Skilled, Business, Unskilled, Student

Marital status — Unmarried, Married

Locality — Rural, Semi urban, Urban

Sociodemographic variable

140 participants were recruited in this study. Age, education, occupation, marital status, and area of residence were the socio-demographic variables recorded and analyzed.

1. Age group was subdivided into 4:
   a) From 16 to 30 years (n=61)
   b) From 31 to 40 years (n= 26)
   c) From 41 to 50 years (n= 32)
   d) From 51 to 66 years (21)

A and b, with p value < 0.05 were statistically significant. Meaning that these age groups had respectively 7.9 and 7.8 chances of presenting themselves for screening.

2. Education

Education was subdivided into, primary, secondary and tertiary education. The later haven been taken for reference, secondary education with a frequency of 13, had a statistically significant value with a p value < 0.05.

Meaning that, the higher one has gone to school, the more the person is susceptible to present herself for cancer screening.

3. Place of residence

Urban dwellers with a statistically significant value of p < 0.05, are more susceptible to to present themselves for screening as compared to persons living in slums and rural areas.

4. Occupation

None of the categories as subdivided here as skilled, business, unskilled /unemployed, had an advantage on the other, although the odds ratio for the unskilled / unemployed was slightly higher.

5. Marital status

The marital status did not have any influence for the person presenting herself for screening or not.

6. Age of first sex

The age of first sexual intercourse had no influence on the person presenting herself for screening.

7. Number of sex partners

The p value for those with more than one sex partners was statically significant with a p value < 0.05 as compared to those who had zero to one partner.

8. The number of pregnancies

There is a statistically significant value of p between pregnancies and screening for cervical cancer.

9. Number of deliveries

There was a statistically significant association between the number of deliveries and cervical cancer screening.

DISCUSSION

In our study, the majority of respondents were aged from 16 to 30 years, followed by the age group of 41to 50. Which is slightly different from the findings of Singh et al, who had 41-50 group, followed by 51-60 (9). This difference could be due to the fact that Buea harbors many tertiary institution and this age group is more conversant with heath challenges.

Our findings are similar to those of Dhodapkar SB et al who reported that,the majority of participants in their study belonged to the age group of 20-24 years (10)

Our findings are however different from those of Belglaiaa E, Souho T, Badaoui L, et al. who had the majority of 41-50 years in her study. This could be explained by the fact that, these women had a comorbidity, which was not the case in our study (11).

There is a good correlation between, high level of education and the probability of coming for cancer screening, according to our study. These findings are different from those of Belglaiaa E, Souho T, Badaoui L, et al (11) and Sara Kebede Tadesse (12). the reason could be that in the two studies cited above, the participants were already sick and were seeking for treatment.

However, our findings on education and cervical cancer in this study are very much in agreement with the works of Khiyali Z (13) , Wihachai et al. (14), Ghahremani et al (15), Rakhshani et al (16) Bebis et al (17) , Shobeiri et al (18),and Swaminathan et al (19)

Many Habitats of slums and rural areas are made of rudimentary, semisolid, thatched or traditionally conceived materials as planks also known as carabot. These are external signs of poverty. In general, these people live below the poverty line as defined by the World Bank, that is with less than 1.9 US dollar /day (20). These conditions are less receptive to preventive measures as they are more focused on how to survive on daily basis. On the other hand, the probability of urban dwellers presenting themselves for screening is statistically significant with a p value < 0.05. this is in accordance with the works of *Jissa V Thu et al (21)*

Occupation is subdivided in our study as skilled, business and unskilled/unemployed. It is understood that people with skilled labour have a higher revenue as opposed to unskilled / unemployed. paradoxically, in this study, the latter had a greater odds to present herself for screening. This could be explained by the fact that, it was a free cancer campaign. our findings are similar to those of Jissa *V Thu et al (21)* .

Marital status

The marital status did not seem to influence participants in this study to present themselves for screening. How ever, some authors say, celibacy, widowhood make women more vulnerable social pressure and do increase their chances of developing a cervical cancer (30, 31, 32)

Age at first sex and number of sexual partners

The age at first sexual intercourse in our study did not influence the participation of the respondent, although there was an increase odd of 0.6. This is not in accordance many findings which put early sexual intercourse as a risk factor for developing cervical cancer. The male factor plays in significant role in the transmission of the HPV virus as the cervix is not yet ripe, it could develop a malignancy (12, 22,23,24,25,26)

Not only did persons with multiple sexual partners have a statistically significant influence to appear in a screening cancer campaign, but they also had an odds ratio of 4.9, meaning that they stand five times the risk of developing a cancer of the cervix. This could be explained by the facts that, the majority of respondents in this study are not married. Added to this, Buea being a cradle of tertiary institutions, participants in this study are much aware of the existence of the cervical cancer.

This is very much in ally with what is found in literature. Early age at at first sexual intercourse and having multiple sexual partners are a risk factors for developing cancer of the cervix (27, 28,29)

CONCLUSION

Despite the fact that cervical cancer is a preventable disease, the toll remains high in the developing world. This study was to find out what are the socioeconomic factors which could influence women to present themselves for cervical cancer screening.

Some of the variables in favor of screening have been identify such as age, the educational level, the residence, the occupation, marital status, age of 1st sexual intercourse, number of sex partners as well as the number of pregnancies and deliveries.

A good understanding of these variables, could help improve on the uptake for primary and secondary measures for prevention, and, help reduce the burden of this disease in our communities.

REFERENCES

1. Effect on an Educational Intervention Based on Protection Motivation Theory on Preventing Cervical Cancer among Margenalized Women in West Iran. Shabnam Malmir, Majid Barati, Ali Khani Jeihooni, Saeed Bashirian, Seyed Mohammad Mehdi Hazavehei. Asian Pacific Journal of Cancer Prevention, Vol 19

2. Kafuruki L, Rambau PF, Massinde A, Masalu N. Prevalence and predictors of Cervical Intraepithelial Neoplasia among HIV infected women at Bugando Medical Centre, Mwanza-Tanzania. Infect Agent Cancer. 2013;8:45.

3. Hemant Kumar Sharma[1,*], Shivani Prashar[2] Impact of socioeconomic risk factors on carcinoma cervix: Hospital based pap smear screening of 2 years in Bihar

4. Kritika Poudel and Naomi Sumi . International Journal of *Environmental Research and Public Health* Analyzing Awareness on Risk Factors, Barriers and Prevention of Cervical Cancer among Pairs of Nepali High School Students and Their Mothers

5. Analyzing Awareness on Risk Factors, Barriers and Prevention of Cervical Cancer among Pairs of Nepali High School Students and Their Mothers

6. Cervical dysplasia. University of Maryland Medical Center. 2015. Available from: https://umm.edu/health/medical/altmed/condition/cervical-dysplasia

7. Cameroon: Human Papillomavirus and Related Diseases, Summary Report 2015 - CMR.pdf. [cited 2020 Feb 10]. Available from: http://www.hpvcentre.net/statistics/reports/CMR.pdf

8. BUEA. [cited 2020 Feb 16]. Available from: http://cvuc.cm/national/index.php/en/about-uccc/the-secretariat/142-association/carte-administrative/sud-ouest/fako/404-buea

9. *Singh S et al.* Original Research Article Awareness about cervical cancer risk factors and symptoms *Int J Reprod Contracept Obstet Gynecol. 2018 Dec;7(12):4987-4991*

10. Dhodapkar SB, Chauhan RC, Thampy S. Knowledge and awareness of cervical cancer and its prevention among nursing staff of a tertiary care teaching institute in South India. Int J Reprod Contracept Obstet Gynecol. 2014;3(4):1056-60. SEP

11. Belglaiaa E, Souho T, Badaoui L, et al. Awareness of cervical cancer among women attending an HIV treatment centre: a cross-sectional study from Morocco. BMJ Open 2018;8:e020343. doi:10.1136/ bmjopen-2017-020343

12. Sara Kebede Tadesse , Socio-economic and cultural vulnerabilities to cervical cancer and challenges faced by patients attending care at Tikur Anbessa Hospital: a cross sectional and qualitative study, BMC Women's Health (2015) 15:75

13. Khiyali Z, Ghahremani L, Kaveh MH, Keshavarzi S (2017). The Effect of an educational program based on protection motivation theory on pap smear screening behavior among women referring to health centers in Fasa. *J Educ Community Health*, **3**, 31-7.

14. Wichachai S, Songserm N, Akakul T, Kuasiri C (2016). Effects of application of social marketing theory and the health belief model in promoting cervical cancer screening among targeted women in Sisaket province, Thailand. *Asian Pac J*

Cancer Prev, **17**, 3505-10.

15. ,, Kaveh MH (2014). Effect of health education based on the protection motivation theory on malaria preventive behaviors in rural households of Kerman, Iran. *Int J Prev Med*, **5**, 463-71.

16. Rakhshani F, Jalilian F, Mirzaei Alavijeh M (2013). Pap smear test among women: an educational intervention based on health belief model. *J Birjand Univ Med Sci*, **20**, 136-43.

17. Bebis H, Reis N, Yavan T (2012). Effect of health education about cervical cancer and papanicolaou testing on the behavior, knowledge, and beliefs of Turkish women. *Int J Gynecol Cancer*, **22**, 1407-12.

18. Shobeiri F, Javad MT, Parsa P, Roshanaei GH (2016). Effects of group training based on the health belief model on knowledge and behavior regarding the Pap smear test in Iranian women: a quasi-experimental study. *Asian Pac J Cancer Prev*, **17**, 2871-6.

19. Swaminathan R, Selvakumaran R, Vinodha J, et al (2009b). Education and cancer incidence in a rural population in south India. *Cancer Epidemiol*, **33**, 89-93. World Bank Sets New Poverty Lines To Measure Poverty, https://www.npr.org/sections/goatsandsoda/2017/10/25/558068646/whats-the-meaning-of-the-world-banks-new-poverty-lines

20. *Jissa V Thu et al*, Socio Demographic and Reproductive Risk Factors for Cervical Cancer – a Large Prospective Cohort Study from Rural India. *Asian Pacific Journal of Cancer Prevention, Vol 13, 2012* 2991

21. Bergmark K, Avall-Lundquivist E, Dickman PW. Patient rating of distressful symptoms after treatment for early cervical cancer. Acta Obstet Gynecol Scand. 2002;81:443–50. [SEP]

22. Corney RH, Everett H, Howells A, Crowther ME. Psychosocial adjustment following major gynaecological surgery for carcinoma of the cervix and vulva. J Psychosom Res. 1992;36(6):561–8. [SEP]

23. Cull A, Cowie VJ, Farquharson D, Livingstone JR, Smart GE, Elton RA. Early stage cervical cancer: psychosocial and sexual outcomes of treatment.[SEP]Br J Cancer. 1993;68:1216–20. [SEP]

24. Eniu A, Carlson RW, El Saghir NS, Bines J, Bese NS, Vorobiof D, et al. Breast health global initiative treatment panel: Guideline implementation for breast healthcare in low and middle-income countries: Treatment resource allocation. Cancer. 2008;113(8):2269–81. [SEP]

25. Hansen RP, Olesen F, Sorensen HT, Sokolowski, Sondergaard J. Socioeconomic patient characteristics predict delay in cancer diagnosis: A Danish Cohort study. BMC Health Services Research. 2008;8:49. [SEP]

26. Hammouda D, Munoz N, Herrero R, Arslan A, Bouhadef A, Oublil M, et al. Cervical carcinoma in Algiers, Algeria: Human papillomavirus and lifestyle risk factors. Int J Cancer. 2005;113:483–9.

27. Bayo S, Bosch FX, de Sanjose S, Munoz N, Combita AL, Coursaget P, et al. Risk factors of invasive cervical cancer in Mali. International Journal of Epidemiology. 2002;31:202–09. [SEP]

28. Kahn JA. An update on humanpapillomavirus infection and Papanicolaou smears in adolescents. Curr Opin Pediatr. 2001;13:303–09. [SEP]

29. Franceschi S, Rajkumar R, Snijders PJ, et al (2005). Papillomavirus infection in rural women in southern India. *Bri J Cancer*, **92**, 601-6.

30. Sauvaget C, Nene BM, Jayant K, et al (2011). Prevalence and determinants of high-risk human papillomavirus infection in middle-aged Indian women. *Sex Transm Dis*, **38**, 902-6.

31. Kaku M, Mathew A, Rajan B (2008). Impact of socio-economic factors in delayed reporting and late-stage presentation among patients with cervix cancer in a major cancer hospital in South India. *Asian Pac J Cancer Prev*, **9**, 589-94.

32. DeGregorio GA, Bradford LS, Manga S, Tih PM, Wamai R, Ogembo R, et al. Prevalence, Predictors, and Same Day Treatment of Positive VIA Enhanced by Digital Cervicography and Histopathology Results in a Cervical Cancer Prevention Program in Cameroon. PLOS ONE. 2016;11(6):e0157319.

33. Enow-Orock G, Mbu R, Ngowe NM, Tabung FK, Mboudou E, Ndom P, et al. Gynecological cancer profile in the Yaounde population, Cameroon. Clin Mother Child Health. 2006;3(1):437–44.

CHAPTER III

DETERMINANTS OF AWARENESS AND KNOWLEDGE ON CERVICAL CANCER AMONG WOMEN IN BUEA- CAMEROON

C. Neh Fru Tassang Andrew, Frederick Nchang Cho, Tassang Thierry and P. Ngum Fru

ACKNOWLEDGMENT

We are thankful to all the women who accepted to participate in this study. We are grateful to all the health personnel/nurses who administered the questionnaires. We express immense gratitude for the great collaboration with the University of Arizona and the Phoenix Medical school for being instrumental in the success of this study.

ABBREVIATIONS

95% C.I - 95% Confidence Interval;

MOH - Ministry of Health;

O.R - Odds Ratio; p, Significance value;

SD - Standard Deviation;

WHO - World Health Organization;

χ^2 - Chi-square.

ABSTRACT

Introduction: The purpose of this study was to assess the knowledge and awareness of cervical cancer among women who came for screening at the regional hospital Buea-South West Region of Cameroon.

Materials and Methods: A descriptive cross-sectional study involving women aged from 16 to 65 years was carried out. A one-day free screening campaign was done at the Buea regional hospital on the 2nd of November, 2019.

Results: The number of sex partners in the last five years had a significant association with the knowledge level. The age, educational status, marital status, age at first sex, and a number of sexual partners for the last past years were associated with knowledge and awareness of cervical cancer screening.

Conclusion: the number of sex partners for the last five years, age, educational level, and marital status were determinants affecting awareness and knowledge in this study. Further studies are needed with larger sample sizes to corroborate or not our findings.

Keywords: Cancer of the cervix, knowledge, awareness, Buea, Cameroon.

INTRODUCTION

More than 85% of cervical cancer worldwide occurs in developing countries [1]. The morbidity and mortality caused by this pathology exert enormous pressure on the fragile health sector of these low-income countries [2].

In developed countries, the health sector is well organized permitting many women to be screened, thus keeping at bay the overwhelming majority of women from the complications of this highly preventable disease [3].

The story is different in Africa South of the Sahara, where, the pyramid is inverted with women coming for consultation at the tail end of the disease, with little or nothing to be done [4].

Cervical cancer, although being the 2nd gynecological malignancy after breast cancer [5], is the 1st cause of death linked to malignancy in women [6].

In Cameroon, about 1993 women develop cervical cancer annually with more than half dying from this disease per year [7]. What could account for this high morbidity and mortality rate among women south of the Sahara in general and Cameroon in particular?

The lack of awareness and knowledge of cervical cancer screening is buttressed by socio-demographic variables [8] such as low socio-economic conditions, ignorance of risk factors such as early engagement in sexual intercourse, multiple sexual partners, early marriages, multiple pregnancies, smoking, low educational level, the lack of knowledge on the manifestations of this disease [9], lack of cervical cancer screening campaigns, cultural beliefs, shyness and discouragement [10].

Prior to the recent creation of the diagnostic and treatment unit of cervical cancer in the Buea Regional Hospital Annex, the hurdles of women with a preliminary diagnosis of cancer were numerous. All suspected cervical cancer patients were referred to the Douala Referral Hospital in the Littoral Region, which is 71.2 Km (1 h 44 minutes) away from Buea. Such referrals had the following odds; transportation, overcrowded cancer services (with only one or two oncologists), and then the French language barrier [11]. Further, patients are given multiple lengthy appointments before being able to meet and consult the specialist [11]. Many of such patients get discouraged, depressed and end up in the hands of herbalists or "Men of God", all of questionable morality, and they finally end up dying without any medical attention [12, 13].

Institutional factors also greatly contribute to the lack of knowledge and awareness, resulting in a high rate of morbidity and mortality. Cancer seems to be a forgotten disease by the public authorities compared to other pathologies which have well-elaborated aggressive awareness campaigns as it is the case with malaria [14] or HIV/AIDS [15]. Added to this, there are barely embryonic structures put in place to take care of cancer [16]. In Cameroon in general, there is no public policy as such to curb this disease which is on the increase. Put aside the Cameroon Baptist Convention (CBC) which is developing specialized units to take care of cervical cancer [17], there are no other stakeholders involved in cervical cancer clinics. Apart from the six referral hospitals of Yaoundé, the political capital, and Douala, the economic capital of Cameroon, the public sector looks desperately as a desert in terms of cervical cancer clinic facilities [16]. In the South West region of Cameroon, there is a small unit in the Limbe Regional Hospital and a maiden service being put in place at the Buea Regional Hospital Annex, thanks to the Cameroon Arizona Partnership program.

The other crux of the matter is the acute shortage of trained personnel, with only a handful of pathologists and oncologists who are all working in the big cities [11]. The situation is not better for other health personnel; nurses, doctors and postgraduate medical doctors specialized in this domain [11].

Studies on the awareness and knowledge [18, 19] of cervical cancer have been carried out in other parts of Cameroon and beyond [6, 20], but none of such studies has been carried out in the Buea Health District.

The objective of this study is to determine factors that can influence awareness and knowledge of cervical amongst women in the Buea health area.

MATERIALS AND METHODS

Study design, sample population, and strategy

This was a hospital-based cross-sectional study carried out on the 2nd of November 2019, in the Buea Regional Hospital which is a government-owned institution of 120 beds. It is an intermediate level health facility that welcomes students of the Faculty of Health Sciences of the University of Buea, as well as students from other health training institutions who come for their clinical internships. Buea and its environ has a population of 200,000 inhabitants [21].

Ethical and administrative clearance

The Institutional Review Board – Faculty of Health Sciences (IRB-FHS) of the University of Buea approved the study and authorizations were obtained from the South West Regional Delegate of Public Health and the Director of the Buea Regional Hospital Annex.

Sampling procedure

Women aged from 21 to 65 years were invited for cervical cancer screening via radio announcements, public banners, posters, and social media platforms.

Peer educators detailly explained the questionnaires and procedures to respondents, as well as assuring them of anonymity and confidentiality. Questionnaires were then administered only to those who consented. Pregnancy women and those with a history of total hysterectomy were excluded from the study.

Sample size determination

The sample size was calculated using the CDC-Epi Info™ 7.2.3.1 StatCalc software as described in another study [8], with the following characteristics: an estimated population size for Buea Health area of 40,000 inhabitants [21, 22], expected frequency of persons living with cervical cancer in Cameroon of 13.8% [23], and an accepted error margin of 5%, design effect of 1.0 and one clusters. Thus, the CDC-Epi Info™ 7.2.3.1 StatCalc estimated the minimum sample size was 182.

Research instrument and Data Collection

The data instrument (paper-based questionnaires) was adapted from a related study [8]. It was prepared in the English language and pre-tested prior to data collection.

The paper-based questionnaire contained sections to capture demographic characteristics, awareness, and knowledge of cervical cancer and cervical cancer screening. Trained peer-educators/ nurses administered the questionnaires. A pilot session of the questionnaire was done prior to the survey in order to ensure that respondents were able to understand it and that questions were interpreted as intended.

Awareness was assessed on a simple Yes/ No question, 'are you aware of cervical cancer screening?'. A negative response was assigned a score of '1'; and a positive response '0'. All of the questions used to assess knowledge of cervical cancer screening in the questionnaire were considered to be true. Knowledge scores for these questions were coded as '0' for a correct response ("True") and '1' for an incorrect ("False"). A composite score was derived for each of the seven questions. A respondent who achieved a composite score of 6 – 7 was considered as highly knowledgeable, 4 – 5 was mediumly knowledgeable and 0 – 3 were lowly knowledgeable.

Study variables

The dependent variables in this study were derived from one question on the awareness of cervical cancer screening and seven questions on knowledge of cervical cancer and its screening. Knowledge of cervical cancer screening was then categorized into three as low, medium, and high. Independent variables were respondents' general characteristics.

Statistical Analysis

Data was captured into Microsoft Excel Office 2018 (Microsoft Inc) and exported to CDC-Epi Info^{TM} 7.2.3.1 (CDC-Epi Info^{TM}, USA) for statistical analysis. Categorical variables are presented as frequency tables and numerical variables as descriptive measures expressed as mean ± standard deviation (SD). The association between knowledge of cervical cancer screening (low/ medium/ high) and demographic characteristics was assessed using bivariate analysis, while awareness (Yes/ No) and demographic characteristics were assessed with bivariate and multivariate logistic regression analyses. Odds ratios (O.R) and Chi-square (χ^2) test were used to compare participants' characteristics with knowledge and awareness of cervical cancer screening multinomial logistic regression was used to identify significant correlates of participants' general characteristics. P-values ≤ 0.05 were considered significant.

Limitations and Strengths of the Study

The data that was acquired from the questionnaire completely depended on self-reported accounts of respondents. However, questionnaires were pre-tested and administered by trained peer-educators or nurses.

RESULTS

A total of 140 consecutively enrolled participants were included in this analysis; their general characteristics are presented on Table 1.

Table 1: Sociodemographic characteristics of study participants

Variable	Subclass	Frequency (%)	95% C.I.
Age groups (Years)	≤ 30	61 (43.6)	35.2 – 52.2
	31 – 40	26 (18.6)	12.5 – 26.0
	41 – 50	32 (22.9)	16.2 – 30.7
	> 50	21 (15.0)	9.5 – 22.0
Education*	Primary	14 (10.1)	5.7 – 16.4
	Secondary	34 (24.6)	17.7 – 32.7
	Tertiary	90 (65.2)	56.6 – 73.1
Marital status*	Unmarried	89 (65.0)	56.3 – 72.9
	Married	48 (35.0)	27.1 – 43.6
Locality*	Rural	29 (20.9)	14.4 – 28.6
	Semi-urban	33 (23.7)	16.9 – 31.7
	Urban	77 (55.4)	46.7 – 63.8
Number of pregnancies*	0 – 4 Pregnancies	108 (82.4)	74.8 – 88.5
	5 – 10 Pregnancies	23 (17.6)	11.5 – 25.2
Age at first sex*	Virgins	4 (3.3)	0.9 – 8.2
	< 20 years	71 (58.7)	49.4 – 67.6
	≥ 20 years	46 (96.7)	29.3 – 47.3
Number of sex partners*	0 – 1 Partner	67 (54.5)	45.3 – 63.5
	> 1 Partner	56 (45.5)	36.5 – 54.7
Occupation*	Skilled	64 (46.0)	37.6 – 54.7
	Business	12 (8.6)	4.5 – 14.6
	Unskilled/ Unemployed	15 (10.8)	6.2 – 17.2
	Student	48 (34.5)	26.7 – 43.1

*Not up to 140 respondents, 95% C.I.; 95% Confidence interval

The ages of respondents ranged from 16 – 66 years with the overall mean (**Error! Filename not specified.** ± SD) age being 35.7 ± 12.6 years. The majority of study participants were young, with43.6% (95% C.I., 35.2 – 52.2) aged 30 years and below, 22.9% (95% C.I., 16.2 – 30.7) between 41 and 50 years,18.6% (95% C.I., 12.5 – 26.0) and 15.0% (95% C.I., 9.5 – 22.0) above 50 years. About two-thirds 90 [65.2% (95% C.I., 56.6 – 73.1)] of the respondents had attended the tertiary status of education, followed by 34 [24.6% (95% C.I., 17.7 – 32.7)] with secondary education and then 14 [10.1% (95% C.I., 5.7 – 32.7)] with primary educational status.

Sixty-four [46.0% (95% C.I., 37.6 – 54.7)] of the respondents were skilled workers (University lectures, lawyers, teachers and nurses), 48 [34.5% (95% C.I., 26.7 – 43.1)] were students, 12 [8.6% (95% C.I., 4.5 – 14.6)] were business women and 15 [10.8% (95% C.I., 6.2 – 17.2)] were either unskilled workers or unemployed (Figure 1)

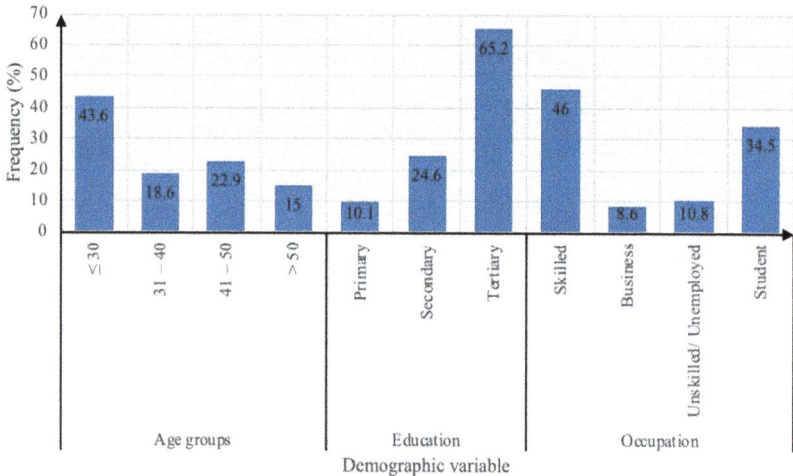

Figure 1: General characteristics of study participants

Reproductive characteristics

More than half of the participants 67/121 (55.4%) had no or one (0 – 1) life, sexual partner, in the last five years, while 3/118 (2.5%) of participants were virgins. One hundred and eight (82.6%) of the 131 respondents who admitted their pregnancy status had had 0 – 4 pregnancies and a fifth (17.6%) had been pregnant 5 – 10 times (Table 1).

Knowledge assessment of cervical cancer screening

Overall, 56/140 [40.0%, (95% C.I., 31.8 – 48.6)] of the study participants were aware of cervical cancer screening. Those who were aware of cervical cancer screening reported that their primary sources of information were from friends/peers 63/140 (45.0%), followed by social media 41/140 (29.3%), radio (10.7%), class teaching (6.4%) and then the television (6.4%) (Figure 3).

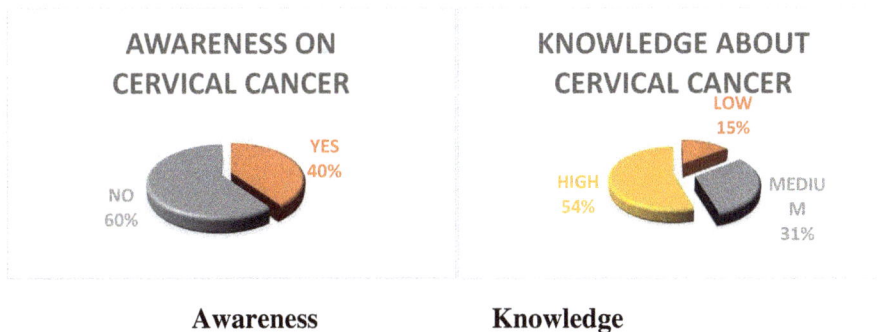

AWARENESS ON CERVICAL CANCER

YES
40%

NO
60%

KNOWLEDGE ABOUT CERVICAL CANCER

LOW
15%

HIGH
54%

MEDIU
M
31%

Awareness   Knowledge

Figure 2: Knowledge levels and awareness of cervical cancer screening

Our results revealed that 20/140 [14.7%, (95% C.I., 9.2 – 21.8)] of the study participants had low knowledge of cervical cancer screening, 42/140 (30.9) had medium knowledge and 74 (54.4%) were highly knowledgeable about cervical cancer screening. The majority of the respondents had good knowledge of cervical cancer as 116/131 (88.6%), 112/126 (88.9%) and 124/127 (97.6%) were aware of the existence of HPV, that HPV increases the risk of CCA and that CCA can be prevented respectively (Figure 2; Table 2). However, only 33/115 (27.8%) of the respondents were conscious of the fact that human papillomavirus could lead to CCA.

Table 2: Awareness and knowledge CCS among study participants (n = 140)

Questions to assess knowledge of CCS†		n	%	95% C.I.
			Frequency of correct responses	
Does HPV exist?		116/131	88.6	81.8 – 93.4
Does HPV increase the risk of CCA?		112/126	88.9	82.1 – 93.8
Can CCA be prevented?		124/127	97.6	93.3 – 99.5
Does lesion treatment prevent CCA?		122/126	96.8	92.1 – 99.1
Is HPV testable?		120/125	96.0	90.9 – 98.7
Does HPV vaccine exist?		88/117	75.2	66.4 – 82.7
Does infection with HPV lead to CCA?		33/115	27.8	19.9 – 36.9
Knowledge of CCS	Low	20	14.7	9.2 – 21.8
	Medium	42	30.9	23.2 – 39.4
	High	74	54.4	45.7 – 62.9
Are you aware of CCS?		56/140	40.0	31.8 – 48.6
Do you know any CCS health unit in the community?		6	4.3	1.6 – 9.1
Previously counseled on CCS?		13	9.3	5.0 – 13.4
Source of CCS information	Class	9	6.4	2.9 – 11.8
	Peers	63	45.0	36.6 – 53.6
	Radio	15	10.7	6.1 – 17.1
	Social media	41	29.3	21.9 – 37.6
	Television	9	6.4	2.9 – 11.8
	Others	3	2.1	0.4 – 6.1

n = number of respondents, % = percentage, CCA = Cervical cancer, CCS = cervical cancer screening, † = the correct response for these questions was 'true'.

Of the 140 respondents, only 13 [9.3%, (95% C.I., 5.0 – 13.4)] had been previously counselled on CCS (Table 2). Six [4.3% (95% C.I., 1.6 – 9.1)] of the 140 respondents accepted knowing of a health unit within the community wherein cervical cancer screening can be carried out, while 97 [69.3% (95% C.I., 60.9 – 76.8)] said, 'I don't know'.

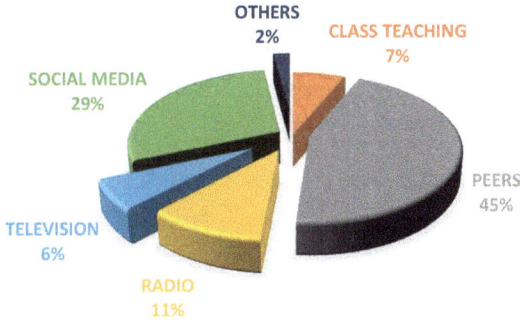

SOURCE OF INFORMATION ON CERVICAL CANCER

OTHERS 2%
CLASS TEACHING 7%
SOCIAL MEDIA 29%
PEERS 45%
TELEVISION 6%
RADIO 11%

Figure 3: Sources of CCS information

Factors associated with Knowledge/ awareness of cervical cancer screening

In bivariate analysis; only the number of sex partners in the last five years was statistically significant ($p = 0.033$) with the knowledge level of cervical cancer screening (Table 3).

Bivariate analysis showed that age, marital status, number of sex partners in the last five years, and occupation were statistically significant ($p < 0.0001$) and associated with the awareness of cervical cancer (Table 4). Multivariable logistic regression showed age and age at first sex were the possible factors influencing the awareness of cervical cancer screening (Table 4).

Table 3: Bivariate analysis for the associations of respondents' characteristics with knowledge of CCS

Variable	Subclass	Low (%)	Medium (%)	High (%)	Total	χ^2 (*p*-value)
Age groups (Years)	≤ 30	5 (25.0)	21 (50.0)	33 (44.5)	59 (43.4)	7.939 (0.243)
	31 – 40	6 (30.0)	5 (11.9)	14 (18.9)	25 (18.4)	
	41 – 50	6 (30.0)	12 (28.6)	13 (17.6)	31 (22.8)	
	> 50	3 (15.0)	4 (9.5)	14 (18.9)	21 (15.4)	
	Total	20	42	74	136	
Education	Primary	3 (15.0)	6 (14.3)	5 (6.9)	14 (10.5)	6.458 (0.167)
	Secondary	8 (40.0)	7 (16.7)	17 (23.6)	32 (23.9)	
	Tertiary	9 (45.0)	29 (69.1)	50 (69.4)	88 (65.7)	
	Total	20	42	72	134	
Marital status	Unmarried	10 (50.0)	28 (68.3)	48 (66.7)	86 (64.7)	2.245 (0.325)
	Married	10 (50.0)	13 (31.7)	24 (33.3)	47 (35.3)	
	Total	20	41	72	133	
Locality	Rural	3 (15.0)	4 (9.7)	21 (28.4)	28 (20.7)	7.823 (0.098)
	Semi-urban	4 (20.0)	9 (21.9)	19 (25.7)	32 (23.7)	
	Urban	13 (65.0)	28 (68.3)	34 (45.9)	75 (55.6)	
	Total	20	41	74	135	
Number of pregnancies	0 – 4 Pregnancies	13 (72.2)	30 (78.9)	62 (87.3)	105 (82.7)	2.813 (0.245)
	5 – 10 Pregnancies	5 (27.8)	8 (21.1)	9 (12.7)	22 (17.3)	
	Total	18	38	71	127	
Age at first sex	Virgins	0 (0.0)	2 (2.9)	2 (3.1)	3 (2.5)	1.067 (0.899)
	< 20 years	12 (63.2)	21 (61.7)	36 (55.4)	69 (58.5)	
	≥ 20 years	7 (36.8)	12 (35.3)	27 (41.5)	46 (38.9)	
	Total	19	34	65	118	
Number of sex partners	0 – 1 Partner	15 (83.3)	18 (48.6)	34 (51.5)	67 (55.4)	6.769 (0.033)*
	> 1 Partner	3 (16.7)	19 (51.4)	32 (48.5)	54 (44.6)	

Occupation						
	Total	18	37	66	121	
Occupation	Skilled	10 (50.0)	18 (42.9)	36 (49.3)	64 (47.4)	11.911 (0.064)
	Business	2 (10.0)	5 (11.9)	4 (5.5)	11 (8.2)	
	Unskilled/ Unemployed	4 (20.0)	0 (0.0)	11 (15.1)	15 (11.1)	
	Student	4 (20.0)	19 (45.2)	22 (30.1)	45 (33.3)	
	Total	20	42	73	135	

*p-values with statistical significance

This study also found that those women who were in the age group of ≤ 30 (16 – 30) years were 18.4 times more likely to be aware of cervical cancer screening than those whose ages were between > 50 (51 – 66) [O.R = 18.4, 95% C.I., 1.8 – 189.8].

Those women who had their first sex at the age of less than twenty years were 4.2 times more likely to be aware of cervical cancer screening as compared to those who had their first sex at more than twenty years old [O.R = 4.2, 95% C.I.: 1.3 – 13.5]. Respondents with the primary school status, unmarried marital status, residents in rural communities, and those with 0 – 1 sexual partners, were more likely to be aware of cervical cancer screening compared to their corresponding counterparts.

Table 4: Bivariate and multivariate associations between respondents' characteristics and awareness of CCS

DV →

| Variable □ | Subclass | Awareness | | | χ^2 (p-value) | p-value | O.R (95% C.I) |
		Yes (%)	No (%)	Total			
Age groups (Years)	≤ 30	11 (19.6)	50 (59.5)	61 (43.6)	23.903 (<0.0001)*	0.01*	18.4 (1.8 – 189.8)†
	31 – 40	12 (21.4)	14 (16.7)	26 (18.6)		0.10	6.0 (0.7 – 51.8)†
	41 – 50	19 (33.9)	13 (15.5)	32 (22.9)		0.05*	7.0 (1.0 – 48.6)†
	> 50	14 (25.0)	7 (8.3)	21 (15.0)		Ref	1.0
	Total	56	84	140			
Education	Primary	7 (12.7)	7 (8.4)	14 (10.1)	1.240 (0.538)	0.20	3.9 (0.5 – 31.1)†
	Secondary	15 (27.3)	19 (22.9)	34 (24.6)		0.70	0.8 (0.2 – 2.8)
	Tertiary	33 (60.0)	57 (68.7)	90 (65.2)		Ref	1.0
	Total	55	83	138			
Marital status	Unmarried	25 (45.5)	64 (78.0)	89 (65.0)	15.366 (<0.0001)*	0.12	2.6 (0.8 – 8.8)†
	Married	30 (54.5)	18 (22.0)	48 (35.0)		Ref	1.0
	Total	55	82	137			
Locality	Rural	10 (18.2)	19 (22.6)	33 (23.7)	0.442 (0.802)	0.58	1.5 (0.3 – 7.1)†
	Semi-urban	14 (25.5)	19 (22.6)	33 (23.7)		0.75	0.8 (0.2 – 2.8)
	Urban	31 (56.4)	46 (54.8)	77 (55.4)		Ref	1.0
	Total	55	84	139			

44

					χ² (p)	p-value	O.R (95% C.I)
Number of pregnancies	0 – 4 Pregnancies	42 (79.2)	66 (84.6)	108 (82.4)	0.629 (0.428)	0.35	0.5 (0.1 – 2.3)
	5 – 10 Pregnancies	11 (20.8)	12 (15.4)	23 (17.6)		Ref	1.0
	Total	53	78	131			
Age at first sex (Years)	< 20	25 (50.0)	46 (64.8)	71 (58.7)	2.646 (0.104)	0.02*	4.2 (1.3 – 13.5)†
	≥ 20	25 (50.0)	25 (35.2)	50 (41.3)		Ref	1.0
	Total	50	71	121			
Number of sex partners	0 – 1 Partner	11 (22.0)	45 (60.0)	56 (44.8)	17.517 (<0.0001)*	0.08	3.1 (0.9 – 10.6)†
	> 1 Partner	39 (78.0)	30 (40.0)	69 (55.2)		Ref	1.0
	Total	50	75	125			
Occupation	Skilled	33 (60.0)	31 (36.9)	64 (46.0)	22.683 (<0.0001)*	0.71	0.7 (0.1 – 3.7)
	Business	9 (16.4)	3 (3.6)	12 (8.6)		0.11	0.1 (0.0 – 1.5)
	Unskilled/ Unemployed	6 (10.9)	9 (10.7)	15 (10.8)		0.69	1.6 (0.2 – 15.8)†
	Student	7 (12.7)	41 (48.8)	48 (34.5)		Ref	1.0
	Total	55	84	139			

*p-values with statistical significance, O.R: Odds Ratio, Ref: Reference, 95% C.I: 95% Confidence interval, † O.R with more likelihood of occurrence.

45

DISCUSSION

Our findings highlight levels of awareness of 40% of cervical cancer and high knowledge (85% of medium and high levels) of cervical cancer screening.

Awareness of cervical cancer screening

In this study, 40% of participants were aware of the fact that cervical cancer exists.

In this study, only 6 (4.3%) of participants could identify a nearby health facility wherein cervical cancer screening is carried out. The paucity of both health personnel specialized in this domain and lack of health structures carrying out preventive tests for cervical cancer is a serious impediment in the fight against cervical cancer. This is in accordance with the works of Gutumo et al in Kenya [24-26] Cancer looks the forsaken child of the health system in Cameroon.

Occupation is vital in the acquisition of awareness and knowledge. Sixty-four (48%) of our respondents were skilled workers (University lecturers, lawyers, teachers, and nurses), the profession had a statistically significant association

($p < 0.0001$) with the awareness of cervical cancer screening. Our results were not however in accordance with the findings of NI Ebu [27] in Ghana. In the latter's study, the modulating circumstance is possibly the fear of stigmatization for being indexed as HIV positive. Contrary to Majetic B et al and Hoque M et al (28,29), we think occupation empowers women, gives them a sense of self-fulfillment, and makes them less dependent on men, giving them autonomy in the decision regarding their health (8).

Age also played a pivotal role in the process of awareness and knowledge. In this study, the age group ≤ 30 years is statistically significant as compared to other age groups and various variables. Cameroon has an essentially young population. The population pyramid of Cameroon in 2018 looked as follows:

0-14 years: 42.15% (male 5,445,142 /female 5,362,166)
15-24 years: 19.6% (male 2,524,031 /female 2,502,072)
25-54 years: 31.03% (male 4,001,963 /female 3,954,258)
55-64 years: 3.99% (male 499,101 /female 524,288)
65 years and over: 3.23% (male 384,845 /female 443,099) [30]

The segment of the population ≤ 24 years represents alone 61.75% of the population.

Our findings look different from those of Ebu in Ghana in which she concluded that older age was a determinant for presentation for cervical screening [27]. The difference further deepens with the works of MJ Park, E-C Park, KS Choi, JK Jun, and H-Y Lee

[31] and E Simou, N Maniadakis, A Pallis, E Foundoulakis, and G Kourlaba [32] in Greece. This could be explained by the structure of their respective populations.

Buea is a cosmopolitan town with 200,000 inhabitants, situated at the foot of Mount Cameroon. This South West regional capital harbors various university institutes, making this town the cradle of learning [21].

Knowledge of cervical cancer screening

Accumulated percentages term respondents in this study as knowledgeable with an accrued score of 85% for both high and mid knowledge on cervical cancer. This figure is higher than the 47% reported in Brazil [33] and lower than the 97.3% reported in Medellin [34]. These differences may be a result of differences in sample design, sizes, and study areas.

Educational level is the driving force for awareness, knowledge, and screening [8]. All authors do agree on this. In this study, this variable is statistically significant. The higher the level of education, the better will awareness, knowledge, and screening. In this study, both secondary and tertiary respondents represent 90% of our sample. Education seems the catalyst that will permit women to judge their health better and make sound decisions accordingly. An educated woman is more cartesian in her analysis as she drifts away from cultural beliefs and myths. the more a woman is educated, the greater the chances of financial autonomy and, she ceases being dependent on men [32, 35-43].

In this study, peers represent 45% of the source of information on cervical cancer. This is in conformity with the work of LG Johnson, A Armstrong, CM Joyce, AM Teitelman, and AM Buttenheim [44]. Social media platforms with a percentage of 25%, came second. This is a powerful method of communication, mostly with the youthful "android generation". Peer influence can go a long way to influence one's behavior. Studies done in Nigeria show that talks given by peers on market places and churches have increased awareness and knowledge in peer groups [45]. Other methods as television, radio, drama have had various fortunes in many African countries, although still being advocated for [46, 47].

In this study, the unmarried variable is statistically significant. NI Ebu [27] also said marital status was not determinant for the intention to be screened for cervical cancer [27]. Many other studies corroborate this; the absence of a relationship between marital status and accepting cancer screening [31, 32, 37]. However, these findings are not in conformity with the works of Lima EG et al, who think that married women do attain antenatal visits and are in a stable and comfortable relationship, this makes them more aware and knowledgeable for cervical cancer [33].

In this study, having a "0–1 sexual partner for the last 5 years" variable was statistically significant. It is thought that a stable relationship, with adequate medical attention, makes the woman more attentive to her health and she is easily predisposed to cervical cancer screening because of the awareness and knowledge she must have acquired thanks be to her medical acquaintances [33].

CONCLUSION

Awareness and knowledge on cervical cancer are modulated by certain variables such as level of education, occupation, age, source of information, marital status, and a number of sexual partners ≤ 1 for the last 5 years. Structural weaknesses of the system as the absence of health structures, lack of medical personnel specialized in oncology, lack of vulgarization of information on cervical cancer by the ministry of public health officials, lack of financial empowerment, and sense of fulfillment of women are strong impediments against awareness and knowledge in the domain of cervical cancer.

LIMITATIONS

- This was a cross-sectional study representing a snapshot of the studied population at a given period in time. It may be difficult to generalize the findings.

- The size of the sample is a self-limiting factor.

- The quality of our sample made mostly of women with a high level of education.

- Demographic data was collected through self-reporting and thus there is a possibility of bias where the respondent provides socially acceptable answers.

RECOMMENDATIONS

- Similar studies should be conducted with larger samples

- The public health authorities should train medical personnel in the field of cancer and empower health structures to carry out common procedures like screening for cervical cancer.

- Simple notions of gynecological cancers should be included in school curricula.

REFERENCES

1. WHO: Cervical Cancer. In.: World Health Organisation; 2018.

2. Kafuruki L, Rambau PF, Massinde A, Masalu N: Prevalence and predictors of Cervical Intraepithelial Neoplasia among HIV infected women at Bugando Medical Centre, Mwanza-Tanzania. *Infect Agent Cancer* 2013, 8(45).

3. NNCTR: Cervical and Breast Cancer Screening Activities in Nepal. In: *Nepal Network for Cancer Treatment & Research*. Cervical and Breast Cancer Screening Activities in Nepal; 2010.

4. Sankaranarayanan R, Budukh AM, Rajkumar R: Effective screening programmes for cervical cancer in low- and middle-income developing countries. *Bull World Health Organ* 2001, 79:954-962.

5. Vaccarella S, Laversanne M, Ferlay J, Bray F: Cervical cancer in Africa, Latin America and the Caribbean, and Asia: regional inequalities and changing trends. *Int J Cancer* 2017.

6. Asonganyi E, Vaghasia M, Rodrigues C, Phadtare A, Ford A, Pietrobon R, Atashili J, Lynch C: Factors Affecting Compliance with Clinical Practice Guidelines for Pap Smear Screening among Healthcare Providers in Africa: Systematic Review and Meta-Summary of 2045 Individuals. *PLoS One* 2013, 8(9):e72712.

7. Bruni L, Albero G, Serrano B, Mena M, Gómez D, Muñoz J, Bosch FX, de Sanjosé S, ICO/IARC.: Human Papillomavirus and Related Diseases in Cameroon. Summary Report 17 June 2019. In. Barcelona, Spain: ICO/IARC HPV Information Centre; 2019.

8. Fru CN, Tassang AN, Cho FN, Tassang T, Fru PN: Socio-economic Determinants Influencing Cervical Cancer Screening in Buea: A Cross-Sectional Study. *International Journal of TROPICAL DISEASE & Health* 2020, 41(11):14 - 22.

9. Joshi M, Mishra SR: Cervical Cancer Screening in Nepal. *Health Prospect Journal of Public Health* 2013, 12(1):18-20.

10. Yamaguchi N, Tsukamoto Y, Shimoyama H, Nakayama K, Misawa S: Effects of peer education interventions aimed at changing awareness of cervical cancer in nursing students. *Niigata J Health Welf* 2011, 11:32–42.

11. Kindzeka ME: Cameroon Doctors Overwhelmed with patients. In. Cameroon: VOA; 2018.

12. Pefok JD: Fake Pastors denounced. In: *Cameroon Postline*. 2018.

13. Nzie F: Poverty, Fake Pastors and Church Businesses. In. Cameroon: Camerounlink Int; 2014.

14. MOH: Plan Stratégique National de Lutte contre le Paludisme: 2014-2018. Ministère de la Santé Publique, Cameroun. In. Edited by Programme Nationale de Lutte contre le Paludisme, vol. 4. Yaoundé: Programme National de Lutte contre le Paludisme; 2014.

15. Mbanya B, Sama M, Tchounwou P: Current Status of HIV/AIDS in Cameroon: How Effective are Control Strategies? *Int J Environ Res Public Health* 2008, 5(5):378-383.

16. Ndom P: Cameroon: Stakeholders commit to intensify cancer screening in local communities. *Journal du Camerouncom* 2020.

17. DeGregorio GA, Bradford LS, Manga S, Tih PM, Wamai R, Ogembo R: Prevalence, Predictors, and Same Day Treatment of Positive VIA Enhanced by Digital Cervicography and Histopathology Results in a Cervical Cancer Prevention Program in Cameroon. *PLoS One* 2016, 11(6):e0157319.

18. McCarey C, Pirek D, Tebeu PM, Boulvain M, Doh AS, Petignat P: Awareness of HPV and cervical cancer prevention among Cameroonian healthcare workers. *BMC Womens Health* 2011, 11(45):45.

19. Heena H, Durrani S, AlFayyad I, Riaz M, Tabasim R, Parvez G, Abu-Shaheen A: Knowledge, Attitudes, and Practices towards Cervical Cancer and Screening amongst Female Healthcare Professionals: A Cross-Sectional Study. *Journal Oncology* 2019, 2019:5423130.

20. Jassim G, Obeid A: Knowledge, attitudes, and practices regarding cervical cancer and screening among women visiting primary health care Centres in Bahrain. *BMC Public Health* 2018, 18(1).

21. NIS.: 2nd Survey on the Monitoring of Public Expenditures and the Level of Recipients' Satisfaction in the Education and Health Sectors in Cameroon (PETS2). In: *Health Component.* Yaoundé National Institute of Statistics; 2010.

22. Nsagha DS, Pokam BT, Assob JC, Njunda AL, Kibu OD, Tanue EA, Ayima CW, Weledji PE: HAART, DOTS and renal disease of patients co-infected with HIV/AIDS and TB in the South West Region of Cameroon. *BMC Public Health* 2015, 15:1040.

23. Nkfusai NC, Cumber SN, Takang W, Anchang-Kimbi JK, Yankam BM, Anye CS, Tsoka-Gwegweni JM, Enow-Orock GE, Anong DN: Cervical cancer in the

Bamenda Regional Hospital, North West Region of Cameroon: a retrospective study. *Pan Afr Med J* 2019, 32(90).

24. Gatumo M, Gacheri S, Sayed AR, Scheibe A: Women's knowledge and attitudes related to cervical cancer and cervical cancer screening in Isiolo and Tharaka Nithi counties, Kenya: a cross-sectional study. *BMC Cancer* 2018, 18(1):745.

25. CRA: Commission on Revenue Allocation. In., 2 edn. Nairobi: Kenya County Fact Sheets; 2013.

26. KIPPRA: Kenya economic report 2013. In. Nairobi: KIPRA; 2013.

27. Ebu NI: Socio-demographic characteristics influencing cervical cancer screening intention of HIV-positive women in the central region of Ghana. *Gynecologic Oncology Research and Practice* 2018, 5(3).

28. Matejic B, Vukovic D, Pekmezovic T, Kesic V, Markovic M: Determinants of preventive health behavior in relation to cervical cancer screening among the female population of Belgrade. *Health Educ Res* 2011, 26(2).

29. Hoque M, Hoque E, Kader SB: Evaluation of cervical cancer screening program at a rural community of South Africa. *East African Journal of Public Health* 2008, 5(2).

30. UNO: World Population Prospects. In. Edited by Department of Economic and Social Affairs PD: UNO; 2019.

31. Park MJ, Park E-C, Choi KS, Jun JK, Lee H-Y: Sociodemographic gradients in breast and cervical cancer screening in Korea: the Korean National Cancer Screening Survey (KNCSS) 2005-2009. *BMC Cancer* 2011.

32. Simou E, Maniadakis N, Pallis A, Foundoulakis E, Kourlaba G: Factors Associated with the Use of Pap Smear Testing in Greece. *J Womens Health* 2010, 19(8).

33. Lima EG, Soares de Lima DB, Miranda CAN, Pereira VSdS, Veríssimo de Azevedo JC, Galvão de Araújo JM, Fernandes TAAdM, Medeiros de Azevedo PR, Fernandes JV: Knowledge about HPV and Screening of Cervical Cancer among Women from the Metropolitan Region of Natal, Brazil. *ISRN Obstet Gynecol* 2013.

34. Hanisch R, Gustat J, Hagensee ME, Baena A, Salazar JE, Castro MV, Gaviria AM, Sanchez GI: Knowledge of Pap screening and human papillomavirus among women attending clinics in Medellın, Colombia. *Int J Gynecol Cancer* 2008, 18(5):1020–1026.

35. Baskaran P, Subramanian P, Rahman RA, Ping WL, Taib NA, Rosli R: Perceived susceptibility, and cervical cancer screening benefits and barriers in Malaysian women visiting outpatient clinics. *Asian Pacific Journal Cancer Prevention* 2013, 14(12):7693–7699.

36. Ezechi OC, Gab-Okafor CV, Ostergren PO, Pettersson KO: Willingness and acceptability of cervical cancer screening among HIV positive Nigerian women. *BMC Public Health* 2013, 13(1).

37. Sichanh C, Fabrice QU, Chanthavilay P, Diendere J, Latthaphasavang V, Longuet C, Buisson Y: Knowledge, awareness and attitudes about cervical cancer among women attending or not an HIV treatment center in Lao PDR. *BMC Cancer* 2014, 14(1).

38. Sudenga SL, Rositch AF, Otieno WA, Smith JS: Brief report: knowledge, attitudes, practices and perceived risk of cervical cancer among Kenyan women. *International Journal Gynecological Cancer* 2013, 23(5).

39. Frank D, Swedmark J, Grubbs L: Colon Cancer screening in African American women. *ABNF J* 2004, 15(4).

40. Gerald EI, Ogwuche CH: Educational level, sex and church affiliation on health seeking behaviour among parishioners in Makurdi metropolis of Benue state. *Infect Dis Rep* 2014, 1(2):311–316.

41. Lee M, Park EC, Chang HS, Kwon JA, Yoo KB, Kim TH: Socioeconomic disparity in cervical cancer screening among Korean women: 1998–2010. *BMC Public Health* 2013, 13(1).

42. Lyimo FS, Beran TN: Demographic, knowledge, attitudinal, and accessibility factors associated with uptake of cervical cancer screening among women in a rural district of Tanzania: three public policy implications. *BMC Public Health* 2012, 12(1).

43. Thomas D: How to reduce maternal deaths: rights and responsibilities. In. London: Department for International Development; 2005.

44. Johnson LG, Armstrong A, Joyce CM, Teitelman AM, Buttenheim AM: Implementation strategies to improve cervical cancer prevention in sub-Saharan Africa: a systematic review. *Implement Sci* 2018(1 - 18).

45. Mbachu C, Dim C, Ezeoke U: Effects of peer health education on perception and practice of screening for cervical cancer among urban residential women in south-East Nigeria: a before and after study. *BMC Womens Health* 2017, 17:1 - 8.

46. Gözüm S, Karayurt O, Kav S, Platin N: Effectiveness of peer education for breast Cancer screening and health beliefs in eastern Turkey. *Cancer Nurs* 2010, 33:213–220.

47. Abiodun OA, Olu-Abiodun OO, Sotunsa JO, Oluwole FA: Impact of health education intervention on knowledge and perception of cervical cancer and cervical screening uptake among adult women in rural communities in Nigeria. *BMC Public Health* 2014, 14.

CHAPTER IV

VACCINATION HESITANCY: THE CASE OF CERVICAL CANCER IN SOME TOWNS OF FAKO DIVISION-CAMEROON

C. Neh Fru, Tassang Andrew, David Greenspan, F. Nchang Cho, Mokake Martin, Joseph Livingstone, Tassang Thierry and P. Ngum Fru, Nembulefac Derick

AUTHORS' CONTRIBUTIONS

This work was carried out in collaboration among all authors. Authors CNF, TA and TT designed the study. Authors FNC and PNF performed the statistical analysis. Authors DG,JL, CNF, TT, TA and FNC wrote the protocol and wrote the first draft of the manuscript. Authors CNF and TA managed the analyses of the study. Authors CNF, TA, FNC and PNF managed the literature searches. All authors read and approved the final manuscript.

INTRODUCTION

The fight against cervical cancer stumbles against resistance accepting vaccines. Vaccination hesitancy is a worldwide phenomenon. it seems this phenomenon is more amplified in Africa. With the advent of COVID 19, many conspiratory theories against all the vaccines have emanated from various quarters. Vaccination against Human Papilloma Virus is no exception to the current dynamics. A study on this topic was carried out in the Fako Division-Cameroon. Some of the reasons why people, for self-reasons, shy away from vaccination against HPV are fear of being Guinee pigs, fear of sterilization of girls, ignorance, doubts about vaccines, religious beliefs, and safety concerns. Some structural causes seem to be the cradle from which vaccination hesitancy is fomented. They are the colonial history, corruption, religious manipulations, and the socio-economic backgrounds of these countries , and mal governance.

The objective of this study is to re-visit the above-mentioned causes and attempt an explanation.

Key-words: vaccination hesitancy, cervical cancer, Fako Division-Cameroon , self-reasons, corruption, religious manipulations, socio-economic background, mal governance, and structural causes.

Reluctance or refusal of vaccines despite their availability is regarded as vaccine hesitancy. It is a worldwide phenomenon to various degrees. The world health Organization classifies it as one of the 10 global health threats in 2019 [1,2].

Why does cancer of the cervix (CC), have a very heavy health burden on the skeletal health systems of low-income countries?

Should a disease be preventable, then surely, cancer of the cervix should be one of them. 99.7 % of cervical cancer (CC) cases are caused by the Human Papilloma Virus (HPV) [1]. The bivalent vaccine, Cervarix ®, potent on HPV 16 and 18, covers 2/3 of all cases of CC [1]. The tetravalent vaccine, Gardasil®, is potent on types 6, 11,16, and 18 [2]. The 9-valent vaccine Gardasil 9® protects against types 6,11,16,18,31,33,45,52 and 58, meaning that the 528.000 worldwide morbid cases and 275000 deaths per annum [3], with 85% of the burden on the developing countries, could be avoided [4].

In the structures of low-income countries in general and Africa south of the Sahara in particular, are there some factors that could account for vaccine hesitancy?

Causes could be subdivided into three categories: structural, individual and governance reasons:

Category 1: STRUCTURAL REASONS:

The economic background :

The scarcity of resources in developing countries accounts for the fact that little attention is paid to social services in general, and cancer in particular *[5,6,7,8]*. Many vaccination and screening campaigns are pilot programs without any continuity *[9,10]*.

Social background:

Sociocultural factors hamper the uptake of vaccines. Because of ignorance, lack of awareness, and knowledge, even the scarce preventive services are underused. lots of religious believes, myths, folktale stories are associated with cervical cancer [10,11]. Powerful antivaccination lobbies do convince people and make them ask the rationale, the effectiveness, and safety of vaccines [11,12]. The consequence is the rejection of vaccines [13].

Historical background

The history of most of these countries plunges into colonization. The majority of low-Income countries are found in Africa south of the Sahara where cervical cancer rates are the highest [3,14,15]. At the helm of most of these states, puppet regimes, answerable to their colonial masters, were installed [16,17]. The primary ambition of these new poorly elected leaders is to mimic their formal masters; the colonizer. The wellbeing of the population seems secondary to them. Their primary ambition is keeping power as long as it is possible and pilling riches above any normal understanding. The bridge of trust between them and the population is not trustworthy. Any social manifestation is looked at with suspicion by the powers that be [16,17]. The resultant consequences are civil strife, socioeconomic instability, corruption, mal governance, an ever-increasing gap of wealth between those governing and the rest of the population, pauperization of the masses, missed priorities, negligence of social services as health and education. [18,19].

The historical peripheral position occupied by Cameroon and Africa should be understood in terms of a metropolis- satellite structures as described by Gunther Frank [20]. the metropolis represented by the developed countries which are the core of the global health system, then the satellite Cameroon, the developing country found at the periphery of the world health system, the metropolis-satellite relationship being unequal [20]. This relationship is exploitative and also creates a dependency and subordinate relation. Increasingly, there is the rejection of the western model of health provision. From this perspective, these are seen as a further strategy to exploit and destroy Africa. The destruction according to this theory will foster the physical occupation of the African territory. this occupation will be a result of the sterilization of all females through vaccination. This point of view is reinforced by the absence or rejection of local health knowledge in the global health system [21]. Some people see a geopolitical strategy in vaccination and asked if Osama Bin Laden was not trapped through vaccination [22,23]. Both vaccines and the western health system are questioned. this has arisen the critical mind of Cameroonians. There is a arise of a critical mindset of Africans vis a vis the global health system [21,24]. According to this point of view, vaccination is another strategy by the former colonial master to subordinate Cameroonians. Not only the vaccines are questioned but also the western model of health. This brings out the level of consciousness of Cameroonians in terms of colonial history which has risen the critical mind of African in terms of health[20,21,25].

Governance

Another major contributor to vaccination hesitancy in Cameroon is linked to governance. According to Cocker [26], " the nature of governance is central because it determines whether the exercise of authority is legitimate". In Cameroon, the issue of poor governance has been addressed [27].

One of our informants expressed the following conspiracy theory: " I am a married person having 2 children all female, and I am 50 years old. I own a shop and I have a GCE A Level. I was in Belgium for some time and came back to Cameroon. I leave in Mile 14. I refused my daughter who is 11 years old to be vaccinated against cervical cancer. The reason is obvious. Don't you know those vaccines are to sterilize young girls so that they should not have children? There is politics in vaccination. There is a hidden agenda behind these vaccines. Do you remember when Americans were in Iraq? They got Sadam Hussein through his children who came for vaccination. The people want to occupy Cameroon".

The second informant had this to say: " I am a 25 years old lady. I have a secondary school level of education. I am a designer and leave in Tiko. All this talk about vaccination is scarring. They will only have to force me out of my house for me to receive it. Our government does not care about her people. Why this sudden concern about vaccination? They provide us nothing, they are corrupt. No water, no electricity. The only thing they have for us is a vaccine. If the president of the republic takes the 1st vaccine and does not die then we will also take it. Let these people not come and depopulate Africa."

In terms of health, this poor governance system has affected and shaped the perception of health issues including vaccination [27,28]. The bridge of trust between the state and the people on whom authority is exercised has affected reactions towards decisions relating to health issues. Population perceives the state as working against the people; so working for the colonial master. the conspiracy theory is thereby reinforced by the absence of trust in those governing. The Question of their legitimacy is expressed by vaccination hesitancy [29,30]. The government does not care about the people, no water, no electricity, why care now in the matter of vaccine? people questioned [27, 29,30]. This depicts the perception grassroots people have of the state in Africa. Their resistance to a vaccine is a subtle way of resisting and fighting authoritative states which are still to attend to some of the increasing challenges like water and electricity plaque in African cities in the 21st century [27]. This resistance to vaccines could also be read under the prism of Africa's resistance to globalization and homogenization of health issues. In other words, resistance to vaccination could be seen as another rejection of colonization manifested through health, a basic human right. Sustainable health will therefore within this context mean the re-humanization of health in Africa. Meaning the creation of schools of medicine with traditional African medicine as part of the curriculum, and respecting the African diversity inclined towards nature. Redressing the power imbalance between the African traditional medicine and the western inputs will improve and greatly scale down vaccination hesitancy.

Gender bias

Women have always been unjustly treated in society from time immemorial. They have not been given equal chances as men. In developed countries, this situation is being addressed. In low-income countries, this phenomenon seems to be on increase aided by the pauperization of the masses. Girls are not given the same opportunities as boys in education. Teenagers are pushed into early marriages. Girls are denied the right of succession, land, and inheritance [20,31]. Women have unequal opportunities for employment and salaries [5]. They are underrepresented in the political and decision spheres [32]. Their pauperization makes them vulnerable economically and they become easy sexual prey for men, and they hardly have access to cancer unit services when they do exist [33,34].

Category 2: INDIVIDUAL CAUSES :

1.Ignorance :

Some groups of people are simply ignorant about the existence and the role of vaccines in preventing diseases.[34,35]

2.Religion :

Economic hardship and the growing pauperization of the masses have led to an untold proliferation of churches [27,28]. Many of these congregations function as sects, with some gurus at their helm [36,37]. Members are brainwashed to the point of dehumanization [7,8,9]. They are made to believe the pastors are custodians of some supernatural powers and are capable of making any type of miracle, including prevention and treatment of any disease. This zombification process puts them at the mercy of these gurus who now dictate the conduct of their followers [37,38,39]. These gurus derive their fame and riches from their followers. These poor people are caged in mental captivity and look as evil some preventive measures and treatment [38,39,40,41,42,43]. these fanatics are the most difficult persons to convince [36,37].

3. Personal beliefs

Some persons do not believe in vaccines and do question their usefulness. To them, nature is powerful enough to stamp out any disease. they asked how Man survived before the advent of vaccination.

Furthermore to them, medicine has made enough progress to put their children at the bay of some ailments. Vaccines are therefore not necessary [34,35].

4. Safety concern

Some people view vaccination under the evil prism. To them vaccination carries along some other diseases to be inflicted on their children, rendering them physically impotent. To some others, this will sterilize their daughters and in the long run depopulate their land with the end objective being the ceasing of their ancestral land by White men [34,35,44,45]

5. Desire of additional info

Amid general mistrust, some " swinging" parents who are ready to vaccinate their children, will like to be convinced about the efficiency of vaccines. They will like to have further details about the vaccines; how they are administered, what are the side effects, and inquire about any long-term complications [46,47,48].

6. Corruption

Corruption be it active or passive has eaten deeply into the fabrics of our society. The government and all its administrative branches are viewed as corrupted [49,50]. While they swim in revolting opulence, the rest of the society crawls in abject poverty [43,44]. Public funds are embezzled at every level of the administration. Kickbacks are the order of the day [51,52,53]. Members of government and functionaries are ready to sign any contract, provided they are given a percentage [49,52,53]. The decisions they take regarding public interest are regarded with suspicion. Amid controversies regarding vaccination, people develop cold feet towards vaccines and they will hardly see anything good as far as vaccination is concerned [52,53,54]. With the financial might commended by pharmaceutical firms, physicians are coopted in the propaganda machinery of these firms. Their neutrality as health experts is questioned by the general population [54,55].

7. Media bombardment

On daily basis, people are bombarded on various media platforms with negative messages against vaccination. Some authors of these messages have a high moral social profile as bishops, academicians, state men, and professors in medicine. These mediatic harassments have a negative impact even on people who could have accepted vaccination [40,41,42,56].

MATERIALS AND METHODS

Study design, sample population, and strategy

This was a community-based cross-sectional study carried out from the 5th to 20th of January 2021, in three communities; Buea, Mutengene, and Tiko in the Fako Division-Cameroon. Buea and its environment have a population of 200,000 inhabitants (NIS., 2010), Mutengene has a population of 32,936 (NIS, 2012) and Tiko has a mainly farming and trading population of 117,883 (Fru et al., 2021).

Ethical and administrative clearance

The Institutional Review Board – Faculty of Health Sciences (IRB-FHS) of the University of Buea approved the study and authorizations were obtained from the South West Regional Delegate of Public Health and the Director of the administration of Atlantic Medical Foundation Hospital – Mutengengene.

Sampling procedure

Persons aged from 15 to 66 years were recruited for the study. Peer educators detailly explained the questionnaires and procedures to respondents, as well as assuring them of anonymity and confidentiality. Questionnaires were then administered only to those who consented.

Sample size determination

The sample size was calculated using the CDC-Epi InfoTM 7.2.3.1 StatCalc software as described in another study[48], with the following characteristics: an estimated population size for Buea Health area of 40,000 inhabitants [49], expected frequency of persons living with cervical cancer in Cameroon of 13.8% [50], and an accepted error margin of 5%, design effect of 1.0 and one clusters. Thus, the CDC-Epi InfoTM 7.2.3.1 StatCalc estimated minimum sample size was 182.

Research instrument and Data Collection

The data instrument (paper-based questionnaires) was adapted from a related study [48].

Trained peer-educators/nurses administered the questionnaires. A pilot session of the questionnaire was done before the survey to ensure that respondents were able to understand it and that questions were interpreted as intended.

Hesitancy towards cervical cancer (CC) vaccine was assessed on the following Yes/No questions, "Will you trust a government's CC vaccine program?", "What will you do if your daughter develops CC?", "Do you believe God can heal CC without medical intervention?".

Study variables

The dependent variable hesitancy, was defined as the proportion of the number of participants who responded with a 'No', to the question " Will you trust a government's CC vaccine program?'', where the numerator comprises all participants who answered 'No' and the denominator comprises the total number of participants in the study.

Independent variables were the demographic characteristics.

Statistical analysis

Data was captured into Microsoft Excel Office 2018 (Microsoft Inc) and exported to CDC-Epi InfoTM 7.2.3.1 (CDC-Epi InfoTM, USA) for statistical analysis. Categorical variables are presented as frequency tables. The association between resistance to CC vaccine and demographic characteristics was assessed using bivariate analysis. The Chi-square ($\chi2$) test was used to compare participants' characteristics with hesitancy to the CC vaccine.

Limitations and Strengths of the Study

The data that was acquired from the questionnaire completely depended on self-reported accounts of respondents. However, questionnaires were pre-tested and administered by trained peer-educators or nurses.

RESULTS

A total of 250 consecutively enrolled participants were included in this analysis; their general characteristics are presented in table 1.

Table 1: Sociodemographic characteristics of studied participants

Variable	Subclass	Frequency (%)	95% C.I.
Age groups (Years)	15 – 20	55 (22.0)	17.0 – 27.7
	21 – 30	62 (24.8)	19.6 – 30.6
	31 – 40	60 (24.0)	18.8 – 29.8
	41 – 50	43 (17.2)	12.7 – 22.5
	> 50	30 (12.0)	8.2 – 16.7
Education	No Formal Education	25 (10.0)	6.6 – 14.4
	Primary	52 (20.8)	15.9 – 26.4
	Secondary	78 (31.2)	25.5 – 37.4
	Tertiary	95 (38.0)	31.9 – 44.3
Sex	Male	78 (31.2)	25.5 – 37.4
	Female	172 (68.8)	62.7 – 74.5
Marital status	Single	97 (38.8)	32.7 – 45.1
	Married	130 (52.0)	45.6 – 58.3
	Divorced	5 (2.0)	0.6 – 4.6
	Widowed	18 (7.2)	4.3 – 11.1
Residence	Buea	82 (32.8)	27.0 – 39.0
	Mutengene	85 (34.0)	28.2 – 40.2
	Tiko	83 (33.2)	27.4 – 39.4

95% C.I.; 95% Confidence interval

The ages of respondents ranged from 15 – 62 years with the overall mean (± SD) age being 33.2 ± 12.7 years. The majority of study participants were in the age group 21 – 30 years, with 24.8% (95% C.I., 19.6 – 30.6), followed by those in the 31 – 40 years age group, 24% (95% C.I., 18.8 – 29.8) and the least being the more than 50 years age group 12% (95% C.I., 8.2 – 16.7). A little more than one-third 95 [38% (95% C.I., 31.9 – 44.3)] of the respondents had attended the tertiary status of education, followed by 78 [31.2% (95% C.I., 25.5 – 37.4)] with secondary education, 52 [20.8% (95% C.I.,

15.9 – 26.4)] with primary and then 25 [10% (95% C.I., 6.6 – 14.4)] with no formal education.

Trusting Cervical Cancer Vaccine related characteristics

Of the 250 participants, only 4 (1.6%) had previously taken the HPV vaccine, and only 70 (29.4%) could trust the vaccine (Table 2). The proportion of participants who will reject the HPV vaccine was 168 (70.6%) of the 250 participants.

Table 2: Hesitancy related characteristics

Variable	Subclass	Frequency	%
Previously taken HPV vaccine	Yes	4	1.6
	No	238	98.4
Trust Government CC vaccination programme	Yes	70	29.4
	No	168	70.6
What do you do if daughter develops CC	Hospital	101	40.4
	Church	63	25.2
	Traditional treatment	86	34.4
Daughter can be next of kin	Yes	30	12.0
	No	220	88.0
Do you believe God can heal CC?	Yes	163	65.2
	No	37	14.8
	Cannot tell	50	20.0
If given only one option, which will you chose?	Church	159	63.6
	Medical Doctor	48	19.2
	Herbalist	25	10.0
	I don't know	18	7.2

Association between Cervical Cancer Vaccine resistant characteristics and patients characteristic

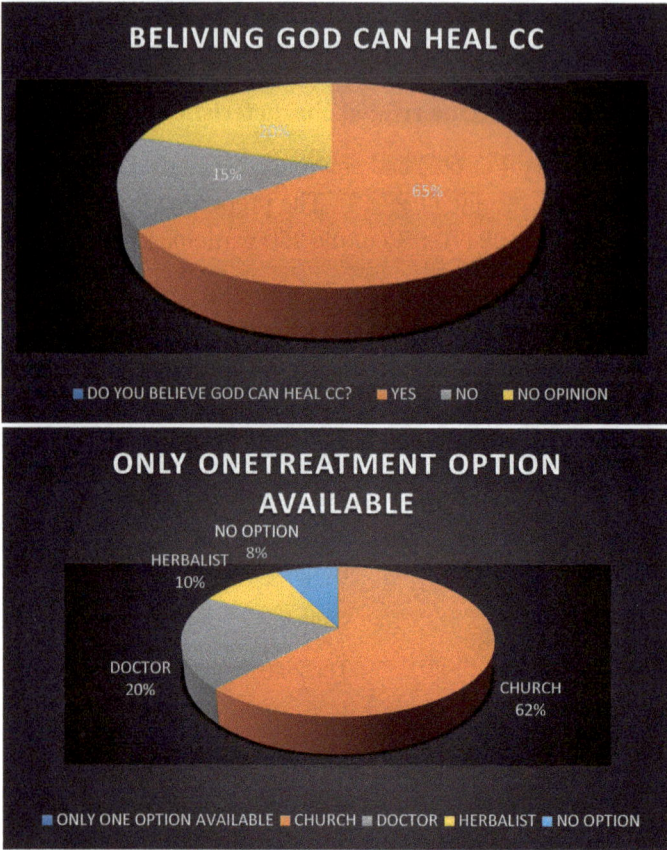

BELIVING GOD CAN HEAL CC

65%

15%

■ DO YOU BELIEVE GOD CAN HEAL CC? ■ YES ■ NO ■ NO OPINION

ONLY ONETREATMENT OPTION AVAILABLE

NO OPTION 8%

HERBALIST 10%

DOCTOR 20%

CHURCH 62%

■ ONLY ONE OPTION AVAILABLE ■ CHURCH ■ DOCTOR ■ HERBALIST ■ NO OPTION

1. BELIEVING GOD CAN HEAL CC

2. IF ONLY ONE TREATMENT OPTION IS AVAILABLE

Chart 1: Asked if they believed God can heal CC, 65% answered by yes, 15% said no, and 20% had no opinion.

Chart 2: If our sample population was given only one treatment option, 62% will prefer the church against 20% for medical treatment. 10% will go for herbalists and 8% were undecided.

Chart 3:71% of our sample does not trust the government in the matter of vaccination against CC. Meaning that only 29% of the population will accept CC vaccination.

Chart 4: 88% of our sample will prefer a male child to be their next of kin.

Bivariate associations between respondents' characteristics and lack of trust

Age and marital status had a significant association (p < 0.05) with trusting the government's decision on CC. All of the participants demographic characteristics except sex and residence had a significant association with, ''what to do if daughter develops CC'' and only age was significantly associated with believing that God can heal CC without medical intervention (Table 3)

Chart 1: Asked if they believed God can heal CC, 65% answered by yes, 15% said no, and 20% had no opinion.

Chart 2: If our sample population was given only one treatment option, 62% will prefer the church against 20% for medical treatment. 10% will go for herbalists and 8% were undecided.

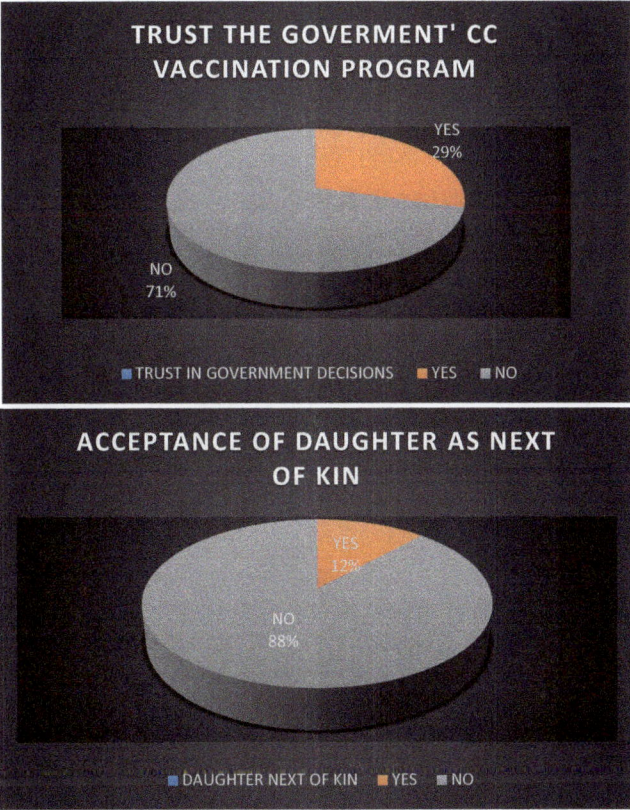

TRUST THE GOVERMENT' CC VACCINATION PROGRAM

YES 29%

NO 71%

■ TRUST IN GOVERNMENT DECISIONS   ■ YES   ■ NO

ACCEPTANCE OF DAUGHTER AS NEXT OF KIN

YES 12%

NO 88%

■ DAUGHTER NEXT OF KIN   ■ YES   ■ NO

3. TRUST IN THE GOVERNMENT CC VACCINATION PROGRAM

4. ACCEPTANCE OF DAUGHTER AS NEXT OF KIN.

Chart 3:71% of our sample does not trust the government in the matter of vaccination against CC. Meaning that only 29% of the population will accept CC vaccination.

Chart 4: 88% of our sample will prefer a male child to be their next of kin.

Bivariate associations between respondents' characteristics and lack of trust

Age and marital status had a significant association (p < 0.05) with trusting the government's decision on CC. All of the participants demographic characteristics except sex and residence had a significant association with, ''what to do if daughter develops CC'' and only age was significantly associated with believing that God can heal CC without medical intervention (Table 3)

Table 3: Bivariate associations between respondents' characteristics and lack of trust

| Variable ↓ | Subclass | Trusting decisions of government on CC vaccination | | | | What will you do if your daughter latter develops CC? | | | | |
		No (%)	Yes (%)	Total (%)	χ^2 (p-value)	Hospital (%)	Church (%)	Tradition (%)	Total (%)	χ^2 (p-value)
Age groups (Years)	15 – 20	9 (5.4)	39 (55.7)	48 (20.2)	129.594 (<0.001)*	20 (19.8)	13 (20.6)	22 (25.6)	55 (22.0)	74.806 (<0.001)*
	21 – 30	27 (16.1)	30 (42.9)	57 (23.9)		29 (28.7)	8 (12.7)	25 (29.1)	62 (24.8)	
	31 – 40	59 (35.1)	1 (1.4)	60 (25.2)		7 (6.9)	31 (49.2)	22 (25.6)	60 (24.0)	
	41 – 50	43 (25.6)	0 (0.0)	43 (18.1)		16 (15.8)	10 (15.9)	17 (19.8)	43 (17.2)	
	> 50	30 (17.9)	0 (0.0)	30 (12.6)		29 (28.7)	1 (1.6)	0 (0.0)	30 (12.0)	
Education	NFE	18 (10.7)	3 (4.3)	21 (8.8)	4.477 (0.214)	3 (3.0)	16 (25.4)	6 (7.0)	25 (10.0)	45.915 (<0.001)*
	Primary	31 (18.5)	19 (27.1)	50 (21.0)		16 (15.8)	20 (31.7)	16 (18.6)	52 (20.8)	
	Secondary	51 (30.4)	23 (32.9)	74 (31.1)		33 (32.7)	6 (9.5)	39 (45.3)	78 (31.2)	
	Tertiary	68 (40.5)	25 (35.7)	93 (39.1)		49 (48.5)	21 (33.3)	25 (29.1)	95 (38.0)	

DV →

Marital status									
Single	61 (36.3)	30 (42.9)	91 (38.2)	10.124 (0.018)*	22 (21.8)	25 (39.7)	50 (58.1)	97 (38.8)	33.243 (<0.001)*
Married	85 (50.6)	40 (57.1)	125 (52.5)		72 (71.3)	28 (44.4)	30 (34.9)	130 (52.0)	
Divorced	5 (3.0)	0 (0.0)	5 (2.1)		1 (1.0)	2 (3.2)	2 (2.3)	5 (2.0)	
Widowed	17 (10.1)	0 (0.0)	17 (7.1)		6 (5.9)	8 (12.7)	4 (4.7)	18 (7.2)	
Total	168	70	238		101	63	86	250	

Believing God can heal cancer without medical attention

		No (%)	Yes (%)	Can't tell (%)	Total (%)	χ^2 (p-value)
Age groups (Years)	15 – 20	2 (5.4)	50 (30.7)	3 (6.0)	55 (22.0)	61.314 (<0.001)*
	21 – 30	12 (32.4)	34 (20.9)	16 (32.0)	62 (24.8)	
	31 – 40	2 (5.4)	45 (27.6)	13 (26.0)	60 (24.0)	
	41 – 50	6 (16.2)	28 (17.2)	9 (18.0)	43 (17.2)	
	> 50	15 (40.5)	6 (3.7)	9 (18.0)	30 (12.0)	
Education	NFE	2 (5.4)	19 (11.7)	4 (8.0)	25 (10.0)	4.678 (0.586)
	Primary	8 (21.6)	36 (22.1)	8 (16.0)	52 (20.8)	
	Secondary	10 (27.0)	53 (32.5)	15 (30.0)	78 (31.2)	
	Tertiary	17 (45.9)	55 (33.7)	23 (46.0)	95 (38.0)	

Marital status					
Single	13 (35.1)	73 (44.8)	11 (22.0)	97 (38.8)	12.101 (0.060)
Married	22 (59.5)	73 (44.8)	35 (70.0)	130 (52.0)	
Divorced	1 (2.7)	3 (1.8)	1 (2.0)	5 (2.0)	
Widowed	1 (2.7)	14 (8.6)	3 (6.0)	18 (7.2)	
Total	37	163	50	250	

*p-values with statistical significance

DISCUSSION

Religion

Our findings are very much per the works of many researchers [36,57,58]

Amidst poverty, people seek solutions in assemblies called "churches". The opening of churches by con-men in searched of riches becomes the order of the day. They are self-aware themselves of titles like Prophets, Bishops, Pastors, Apostles, Papa, "Man of God" etc. Aided by the morose economic atmosphere biting hard into the fabrics of the society, these gurus set out to preach the " gospel of prosperity". In the name of " miracles", people in search of a solution to their problems flock in their numbers into these churches [60,61]. They become the fertile ground on which the gurus build their riches. As much as Jesus Christ fed a crowd of 5000 people, nowadays 5000 people feed a single person. Keeping these people as " mental slaves" becomes an absolute task for the gurus [36, 58].

The methodological mental dehumanizing procedure is systematically put in place. The poor followers are expunged of their personality [57,58]. They are transformed into living -deads, zombies who are remote-controlled by the gurus of the so-called churches. The zombification process is so profound that "these wretches on earth'' skid away from any rational behavior. they worked and act according to the dictates of " their "Apostles, Prophets, Bishops, Pastors, Papa, Man of God'. The flocks are made to believe that their leaders have mystical powers to find solutions and treat among others any type of disease, cancer inclusive. In their illusion, they believe cancer could be treated by prayers in the name of "miracle", and nothing contrary to this can dissuade them [36,61,63].

These people are transformed into "mystical-religious" beings. Vaccination is regarded as evil with devastating effects. The prophets make them believe the optimum protection are prayers alone [36,64].

Politico - corruption

Fueled by the current controversies around Covid-19, a stiff resistance has developed against CC vaccination [65,66,67]. With many authors, we agree that many of those at the helm of the state are regarded as corrupted [47,50,68]. Their decisions are influenced by what they can gain personally [51,52,53]. Abnegation is kilometers away from them. Public contracts are signed depending on how handsome are the kick-backs. the prisons are full of top government officials who have embezzled huge sums of public money [68,69]. The denizens are bewildered and look at those governing them as scavengers, ready to sacrifice them at the least opportunity. In our study, 71%

of our sample population will not accept vaccination against CC. The reasons are multiple. People fear being Guinee picks in the hands of powerful firms who have bought over those governing them [34,35,44]. Some fear it is a ploy to render their loved ones barren and subsequently wipe them from the surface of the earth. Some others think the side effects will be disastrous [33,34,335]. For all these reasons, people develop cold feet towards vaccination and look for other avenues to protect themselves.

Personal conviction

In our study, the 8% of our sample size who will rather go to herbalists for treatment are probably, people who do not believe in modern methods of prevention and treatment of CC or who have some concern with the safety of a treatment or desire some additional information about CC treatment.

This group of persons individually or aided by herbalists say vaccines are not necessary because nature has a response to every situation. They believe in natural immunity. To them,

vaccination is equivalent to introducing a foreign object into one's system which is not advisable [34,35, 46,47].

Gender bias

The traditional society the world over is full of bias against women, Africa is no exception. Women are denied some basic rights rending them vulnerable to some disease [30,31]. Our study is following the works of many authors [30,31,71]. Just 12% of our sample will make their daughter next of kin. Many researchers agree on the fact that capacitating the woman financially, academically, professionally will enhance their autonomy and keep them at the bay of dependency. They can take rational decisions concerning their health and act accordingly.

CONCLUSION

Vaccination hesitancy does not seem to be an isolated phenomenon. Its causes could be explained at three main levels. The first level or structural causes are the colonial backgrounds of these countries, the corruption of the leaders, the vulnerable economic background, and gender bias. At the individual level, some of the reasons are ignorance, personal beliefs, desire for more information, religious dehumanization, influence by the media, and safety concern. Mal governance is imbedded in the cupidity of those at the helm of the country. Taking into consideration the above-mentioned causes will help Understanding better the phenomenon of vaccination hesitancy.

REFERENCES

1. Sarah Finocchario-Kessler, Catherine Wexler, May Maloba, Natabhona Mabachi, Florence Ndikum-Moffor & Bukusi . Cervical cancer prevention and treatment research in Africa: a systematic review from a public health perspective. *BMC Women's Health* volume 16, Article number: 29 (2016)

2 Mamsau Ngoma and Philippe Autier. Cancer prevention: cervical cancer. Ecancermedicalscience. 2019; 13: 952.Published online 2019 Jul 25. doi: 10.3332/ecancer.2019.952

3. Kafuruki L, Rambau PF, Massinde A, Masalu N. Prevalence and predictors of Cervical Intraepithelial Neoplasia among HIV infected women at Bugando Medical Centre, Mwanza-Tanzania. Infect Agent Cancer. 2013;8:45.

4. Franco EL, Duarte–Franco E, Ferenczy A. Cervical cancer: epidemiology, prevention and the role of human papillomavirus infection. CMAJ. 2001;164:1017–25.

5. Shrestha AD, Neupane D, Vedsted P, Kallestrup P. Cervical cancer prevalence, incidence and mortality in low and middle income countries: a systematic review. *Asian Pac J Cancer Prev*. 2018;19(2):319-324.

6. Vaccarella S, Lortet-Tieulent J, Plummer M, Franceschi S, Bray F. Worldwide trends in cervical cancer incidence: impact of screening against changes in disease risk factors. *Eur J Cancer*. 2013;49(15):3262-3273.

7. Holme F, Kapambwe S, Nessa A, Basu P, Murillo R, Jeronimo J. Scaling up proven innovative cervical cancer screening strategies: challenges and opportunities in implementation at the population level in low- and lower-middle-income countries. *Int J Gynaecol Obstet*. 2017;138(suppl 1):63-68.

8. World Health Organization. *Assessing National Capacity for the Prevention and Control of Noncommunicable Diseases: Report of the 2017 Global Survey*. Geneva, Switzerland: World Health Organization; 2018. https://apps.who.int/iris/bitstream/handle/10665/276609/9789241514781 -eng.pdf. Accessed December 12, 2019.

9. Institute for Health Metrics and Evaluation. *Financing Global Health 2018: Countries and Programs in Transition*. Seattle, WA: Institute for Health Metrics and Evaluation; 2019. http://www.healthdata.org/sites/default/files/files/policy_report/FGH/201 9/FGH_2018_full-report.pdf. Accessed September 28, 2019.

10. Weyinshet Gossa , Michael D Fetters. How Should Cervical Cancer Prevention Be Improved in LMICs?AMA J Ethics. 2020 Feb 1;22(2):E126-134. doi: 10.1001/amajethics.2020.126.

11. Kabakama S, Gallagher KE, Howard N, et al. Social mobilisation, consent and acceptability: a review of human papillomavirus vaccination procedures in low and middle-income countries. *BMC Public Health*. 2016;16(1):834.

12. International Agency for Research on Cancer, World Health Organization. Cancer fact sheets: cervix uteri. http://gco.iarc.fr/today/data/factsheets/cancers/23-Cervix-uteri-fact-sheet.pdf. Published March 2019. Accessed April 10, 2019.

13. Lane S, MacDonald NE, Marti M, Dumolard L. Vaccine hesitancy around the globe: analysis of three years of WHO/UNICEF Joint Reporting Form data-2015-2017. *Vaccine*. 2018;36(26):3861-3867.

14. WHO: Cervical Cancer. In.: World Health Organisation; 2018.

15. Shabnam M, Barati M, Jeihooni AK, Bashirian S, Hazavehei SMM. Effect on an educational intervention based on protection motivation theory on preventing cervical cancer among marginalised women in West Iran. Asian Pac J Cancer Prev. 2018;19(3):755-61.

16. What is the French Colonial Tax?. Angeline Mbogo. Afritech News. July 7, 2020September 15, 2020. https://afritechnews.com/french-colonial-tax/

17. Mawuna Remarque KOUTONIN .France/Afrique : 14 African Countries Forced by France to Pay Colonial Tax For the Benefits of Slavery and Colonization . MediaPart. Dec. 2020 https://blogs.mediapart.fr/jecmaus/blog/300114/franceafrique-14-african-countries-forced-france-pay-colonial-tax-benefits-slavery-and-colonization

18. BBC World Service. The story of Africa: African history from the dawn of time. http://www.bbc.co.uk/worldservice/africa/features/storyofafrica/index.sht ml. Accessed August 15, 2019.

19. Indice de perception de la corruption 2018 : Transparency International pointe la faiblesse des institutions africaines. *Fatoumata Diallo*. Jeune Afrique Business+. 12 novembre 2019.

20. Gunther Frank. Capitalism and Underdevelopment in Latin America New York: Monthly Review Press 1967, revised ed. 1969, London: Penguin Books 1971

21. Savanna L. Carson ,Fabrice Kentachime, Cyrus Sinai, Elizabeth A. Van Brian L. Hilary A. Godwin Cole & Hilary A. Godwin. Health Challenges and Assets of Forest-Dependent Populations in Cameroon. https://link.springer.com/oscar-static/images/springerlink/svg/springerlink-253e23a83d.svg . 21 May 2019

22. https://www.theguardian.com/world/2011/jul/11/cia-fake-vaccinations-osama-bin-ladens-dna

23. https://www.nationalgeographic.com/science/article/150225-polio-pakistan-vaccination-virus-health

24. Ali Arazeem Abdullah. Trends and Challenges of Traditional Medicine in Africa. Afr J Tradit Complement Altern Med. 2011; 8(5 Suppl): 115–123. 2011 Jul 3. doi: 10.4314/ajtcam.v8i5S.5

25. Sara Cooper,Cornelia Betsch, Evanson Z. Sambala, Nosicelo Mchiza, and Charles S. Wiysonge. Vaccine hesitancy – a potential threat to the achievements of vaccination programmes in Africa. Hum Vaccin Immunother. 2018; 14(10): 2355–2357. 2018 May 22. doi: 10.1080/21645515.2018.1460987

26. Chester A. Crocker . African Governance: Challenges and Their Implications.African Governance: Challenges and Their Implications. GOVERNANCE IN AN EMERGING NEW WORLD, Winter Series, Issue 119. January 14, 2019

27. Achille Mbembe. In Cameroon, change will not come from the ballot box. Jeune Afrique. October 27, 2018

28. https://theconversation.com/what-tanzanias-covid-19-vaccine-reluctance-means-for-its-citizens-and-the-world-155310

29. Tahiru Azaaviele Liedong. African citizens have good reasons to be fed up with their politicians. The Conversation.July 17 2017.

30. Claire Felter. Africa leaders for life. https://www.cfr.org/backgrounder/africas-leaders-life. *June 30, 2020*

31. How African policies are promoting gender equality in education.Hendrina Chalwe Doroba. Forum for African Women Educationalists (FAWE). October 11, 2017 .
https://www.globalpartnership.org/blog/how-african-policies-are-promoting-gender-equality-education.
https://faculty.wcas.northwestern.edu/~sjv340/roots_of_gender_inequality.pdf

32. Gumisai Mutume. African women battle for equality. Africa Renewal. July 2005

33. WOMEN IN DEVELOPING COUNTRIES REPORT. Flash Eurobarometer 372. March 2013.

34. Neh Fru ,Tassang Andrew et AL. Determinants of Awareness and Knowledge on Cervical Cancer among Women in Buea- Cameroon . International Journal of Research and Reports in Gynaecology . 3(3): 1-14, 2020; Article no.IJRRGY.61689

35. Gallagher KE, LaMontagne DS, Watson-Jones D. Status of HPV vaccine introduction and barriers to country uptake. *Vaccine.* 2018;36(32)(pt A):4761-4767.

36. Maryam Yahya. Polio vaccines—"no thank you!" barriers to polio eradication in Northern Nigeria *African Affairs*, Volume 106, Issue 423, April 2007, Pages 185–204, https://doi.org/10.1093/afraf/adm016

37. Chephra McKee, and Kristin Bohannon. Exploring the Reasons Behind Parental Refusal of Vaccines. J Pediatr Pharmacol Ther. 2016 Mar-Apr; 21(2): 104–109. doi: 10.5863/1551-6776-21.2.104

38. Pefok JD. Fake pastors denounced. In: Cameroon Postline;2018.

39. Nzie F. Poverty, fake pastors, and church businesses. In.Cameroon. Camerounlink Int; 2014.

40. Gordana Pelčić et al.Religious exception for vaccination or religious excuses for avoiding vaccination. Croat Med J. 2016 Oct; 57(5): 516–521.

41. Falade, Bankole Adebayo, Vaccination Resistance, Religion and Attitudes to Science in Nigeria. Phd thesis. January 2014. https://core.ac.uk/download/pdf/46517693.pdf

42. CAMEROON: Catholic Bishops Express Worry on Cervical Cancer Vaccine. Catholic information service for Africa. November 10,2020. http://cisanewsafrica.com/cameroon-catholic-bishops-express-worry-on-cervical-cancer-vaccine/

43. African Church voices "doubts" over cervical cancer vaccine. La Croix International. Dec, 22, 2020. https://international.la-croix.com/news/ethics/african-church-voices- doubts-over-cervical-cancer-vaccine/13314.

44. Cameroon: Obala Diocese prohibits administration of cervical cancer vaccine on girls. Journal du Cameroun.com. 20.10.2020. https://www.journalducameroun.com/en/cameroon-obala-diocese-prohibits-

45. VanderbiltFaculty & Staff Health and Wellness.Immunizations and Religion. https://www.vumc.org/health-wellness/news-resource-articles/immunizations-and-religion.

46. JEAN-PHILIPPE CHIPPAUX. Africa, Big Pharma's guinea pig. Le Monde Diplomatique. June 2005. https://www.mondediplomatique.fr/2005/06/CHIPPAUX/12513

47. Pierre Bienvault . Faced with anti-vaccines, Inserm counter-attacks. La Croix. 2/18/2017 https://www.la-croix.com/Sciences-et-ethique/Sante/INFOGRAPHIE-Face-anti-vaccins-lInserm-contre-attaque-2017-12-18-1200900421

48. Think Global Health. Vaccine Hesitency, an Escalading Danger in Africa. https://www.thinkglobalhealth.org/article/vaccine-hesitancy-escalating-danger-africa.

49.Mary Amuyunzu-Nyamongo .Reasons for vaccine Non-Acceptance in the African   Region. https://www.who.int/immunization/research/meetings_workshops/non_accepta nce_africa_amuyunzun_ivirac_jun14.pdf

50.Gallagher KE, LaMontagne DS, Watson-Jones D. Status of HPV vaccine introduction and barriers to country uptake. *Vaccine.* 2018;36(32)(pt A):4761-4767

51.Global corruption barometer Africa 2019: citizens' views and experiences of corruption. https://www.transparency.org/en/publications/gcb-africa-2019#

52.La corruption, toujours, au Cameroun. https://www.dw.com/fr/la-corruption-toujours-au-cameroun/a-49558429

53.1 in 4 Africans had to pay a bribe to access public services last year. https://www.weforum.org/agenda/2019/07/africa-corruption-bribe-economy/

54. *Fatoumata Diallo.* Indice de perception de la corruption 2018 : TransparencyInternational pointe la faiblesse des institutions africaines. Jeune Afrique Business+. 12 novembre 2019.

55.GERDDES Cameroun. De la corruption au Cameroon. FRIEDRICH EBERT STIFTUNG. Juin 1999.

56.Amber Hsiao ,Verena Vogt, Wilm Quentin . Effect of corruption on perceived difficulties in healthcare access in sub-Saharan Africa. Plos One. Published: August 21, 2019 . https://doi.org/10.1371/journal.pone.0220583

57.Global Health Research in an Unequal World. EVERYBODY'S CORRUPT: UNDERSTANDING SUSPICION IN MEDICAL RESEARCH. https://www.ncbi.nlm.nih.gov/books/NBK458761/

58.Rozem Morgat. Comment les anti-vaccins squattent les réseaux sociaux . Liberation. 11 juillet 2017. https://www.liberation.fr/france/2017/07/11/comment-les-anti-vaccins-squattent- les-reseaux-sociaux_1583123

59.Neh Fru C, Tassang Andrew, Frederick Nchang Cho, Tassang Thierry and P. Ngum Fru. Determinants of awareness and knowledge on cervical cancer among women in Buea- Cameroon. International Journal of Research and Reports in Gynaecology. 2020;3(3):1-14.

60.NIS. 2010. 2nd Survey on the Monitoring of Public Expenditures and the Level of Recipients' Satisfaction in the Education and Health Sectors in Cameroon (PETS2). *Health Component.* 2 ed. Yaoundé National Institute of Statistics.

61.NKFUSAI, N. C., CUMBER, S. N., TAKANG, W., ANCHANG-KIMBI, J. K., YANKAM, B. M., ANYE, C. S., TSOKA-GWEGWENI, J. M., ENOW-OROCK, G. E. & ANONG, D. N. 2019. Cervical cancer in the Bamenda

Regional Hospital, North West Region of Cameroon: a retrospective study. *Pan African Medical Journal, 32.*

62. Nzie F. Poverty, fake pastors, and church businesses. In.Cameroon. Camerounlink Int; 2014.

63. https://www.facebook.com/Stopfakepastors/posts/fraudfake-miracles-cameroon-shuts-down-100-pentecostal-churches-cameroons-presid/1686376904972768/

64. https://mimimefoinfos.com/buea-pastor-fails-to-escape-custody-after-dubbing-people-of-millions-of-fcfa/

65. https://www.journalducameroun.com/en/cameroon-fake-pastor-arrested-for-raping-30-young-girls-in-yaounde/

66. https://cameroonpostline.com/fake-pastors-denounced/%E2%80%8B

67. https://mimimefoinfos.com/buea-pastor-fails-to-escape-custody-after-dubbing-people-of-millions-of-fcfa/

68. https://theconversation.com/three-major-scientific-controversies-about-coronavirus-144021

69. https://pubmed.ncbi.nlm.nih.gov/32817231/

70. https://jme.bmj.com/content/46/7/419

71. https://www.jeuneafrique.com/339468/politique/cameroun-operation-epervier-poids-lourds-restent-prison/

72. https://www.jeuneafrique.com/339468/politique/cameroun-operation-epervier-poids-lourds-restent-prison/

73. The Roots of Gender Inequality in Developing Countries .Seema Jayachandran. Annual Reviews of economics. February 2015.

CHAPTER V

VACCINATION AGAINST CERVICAL CANCER: PROFILE OF ACCOMMODATING PARENTS AND SOME SUGGESTIONS TO OVERCOME HESITANCY AGAINST VACCINATION

Tassang Andrew, Halle Ekane G E, C. Neh Fru, Frederick Nchang Cho, Tassang Thierry, T. Palle Ewane P. Ngum Fru Daniel Ndongo, W. Ndakason, G. Ncham, and Tangui Gracious

ABSTRACT

Cancer of the cervix is a preventable disease. methods of prevention are divided into primary, secondary, and tertiary. Vaccination falls into the primary methods. Despite the avoidable nature of this disease, there is a growing hesitancy in society to allow girls to be vaccinated. Sensitization by the public authorities, financial empowerment of women, and level of education seem crucial to increase the uptake of vaccination against the Human Papilloma Virus.

Key-words: prevention, vaccination, cervical cancer, Human Papilloma Virus, hesitancy

INTRODUCTION

Far from being a thunder striking under a serene blue sky, cervical cancer is rather an old diesel lorry climbing a stiff slope at a chameleon's pace, giving ample time to curb the disease at its very beginning. Despite the annual figures of 528000, with more than 266000 fetal cases [1], this disease remains essentially preventable [2]. Carcinoma of the cervix is the prototype of disease which portraits the gigantic gap which exists between the health systems of the developed and the developing countries [3,4].

The developing world alone accounts for 85 % of all the cases, with Africa south of the Sahara paying a heavy toll [5].

Human papillomavirus (HPV) infection is by excellence a sexually transmissible disease, with about 75% of sexually active women at risk of contracting it during their active lifespan [6].

The primary preventable method is vaccination among others and the secondary preventable method is cervical cancer screening and treatment of precancerous lesions.

The risk factors such as early sexual encounter, early marriage, multiple sexual partners for both members of a couple, polygamy, sexually transmissible diseases, Nonuse of

78

preservative during sexual intercourse, low educational level, lack of awareness, poor economic status, cigarette smoking, and Absence of preventive methods are generally not known to our population ([7].

Could the background of our countries account for what is being observed?

The economic background:

Most low-income countries have limited resources, priorities are elsewhere. Extremely marginal resources and attention are allocated to the fight against cancer[8,9,10,11]. With the lack of funds, many screening exercises are pilot programs [12,13]. scarce resources are directed for cervical cancer prevention. The disparity in funding is abyssal. 81% of funding to fight against cervical cancer is benefited by the high-income countries with only 16.6 % of the global population. [14]

Social background:

Sociocultural factors also have an impact on the prevention of cervical cancer, resulting in low uptake of vaccines. Preventive services though scarce, are underused because of a lack of awareness and knowledge about cervical cancer. This disease carries a stigma because of its anatomic site, stories associated with the disease, and religious beliefs [15].

There is existing in the communities of powerful lobbies against vaccination, questioning the rationale, the safety, and the effectiveness of vaccines [16], making people develop a strong sense of resistance against vaccines [17].

Prevention of cervical cancer

Prevention against cervical cancer is divided into three: primary, secondary, and tertiary.

Primary methods are abstinence from sex, fidelity to one partner, male circumcision as it reduces the risk of HPV carried by the male partner, barrier methods, and vaccination [18, 19].

Secondary preventive methods are based on screening tests and the immediate treatment of precancerous lesions. They are Pap smear, visual inspection methods (visual inspection with 3-5% acetic acid [VIA]/ visual inspection with Lugol iodine [VILI]), and HPV DNA rapid results testing. These tests can help curb about 80% of cervical cancer [20].

The tertiary method of prevention of cervical cancers is made of the treatment of early precancerous lesions. They consist of cryotherapy, loop electrosurgical excision procedure (LEEP), and cold-knife conization [21,22,23,24,25].

Vaccination against HPV

The role of vaccination is depicted by the fact that, despite the overlapping nature of preventive methods for fighting against STDs and HPV, the transmission of HPV remains high [7]. Furthermore, 75% of sexually active women will be confronted with HPV infection, at some point in their lives [26].

Three types of vaccines are present on the market, namely [7] :

The 9-valent vaccine, known as Gardasil 9® , efficient against HPV types 6,11,17,19,32,34,46,53,59.

The quadrivalent vaccine, commercialized as Gardasil®, efficient against types 6,11,17, and 19 of HPV.

And lastly, the bivalent type bearing the commercial name of Cervarix®, potent against types 16 and 18 of HPV.

99.7 % of cervical cancers (CA) are caused by HPV [28] and types 16 and 18, are responsible for 2/3 of premalignant lesions of the cervix [28, 29].

WHO recommends vaccination before sexual exposure. The vaccine is administered to girls age 9 to 14 years in two doses. The second dose is given 6 months away from the 1st dose. For girls beyond 15, a 3rd dose is given at 12 months [7].

Not only Vaccines can prevent more Than 95% of HPV 16 and 18 infections, but it also cross-protects against other types of viruses responsible for anogenital warts; types 6 and 11 [30]. Many studies carried out around the world have proven the efficiency of vaccination against HPV, with a sharp reduction of preinvasive disease [31].

The safety of all the vaccines is assured according to the WHO [32].

Despite the recommendation of WHO, many African countries because of economic reasons, are unable to integrate into their national vaccination programs, vaccination against HPV [33] . Added to this, people not only question the usefulness of HPV vaccines, but they go further to interrogate their safety, and above all, the malignant intentions of these vaccines [34,35,36].

The objective of this study is to draw the profile of parents who bring their children for vaccination despite the societal bias against cervical cancer vaccination.

MATERIALS AND METHODS

Study design setting and strategy

It was a pilot campaign, with 100 doses of Cervarix®, provided by the Cameroon – Arizona partnership program (CAP). The supplementary 1 dose was given by the Baptist hospital in Mutengene.

Parents were invited via social media campaigns, radio announcements, posters, and banners, to bring along for vaccination their daughters aged between 9-14 years.

We soon realize hostile messages directed at vaccination against HPV pupping here and there on various platforms we used to advertise this campaign. Using the same media, we resorted to addressing the peoples' preoccupations, and also, we explained the advantages of having their daughters vaccinated. The negative messages kept on coming. We now decided to call on the phone some of the parents, so we could explain the benefits of having their offspring vaccinated. We went further, meeting parents and having a one on one discussion, trying to persuade them on the effectiveness and safety of vaccination against HPV. Some of the parents who got convinced said, they will do so because of the confidence they have in the vaccination team. The campaign was ignited in the Buea regional hospital, which is an intermediate government-owned health facility with a capacity of 120 beds. It serves the 200.000 inhabitants of Buea. it is the referral health structure for Buea and its environs [37].

On Saturday the 6th of May 2019, at the end of the day, only 65 girls were brought for vaccination. The second part of this exercise was taken to a different town, Mutengene some 15 km south of Buea. The Baptist hospital Mutengene has a capacity of 151 Beds and is the biggest health structure in that Health Area with its 47.500 Inhabitants. This hospital receives clients from other regions and even from foreign countries [38].

Since the population of this area is predominantly of the Christian faith, we took advantage of the next day which was a Sunday to relaunch a new campaign in churches in Mutengene. The following day, Monday was again used for sensitization. On Tuesday, the 37 remaining doses were administered in the Baptist hospital Mutengene. The second doses of vaccines were administered 6 months later.

Ethical and administrative clearance

The ethical clearance was obtained from the review board of the Faculty of Health Sciences, and the administrative authorizations were obtained from the South West Regional Delegate of Public Health and the director of Buea regional hospital.

Study population and procedure

All accompanying parents were lectured on the advantages of having their daughter (s) vaccinated. An open questions and answers session ensued. The procedure of vaccination was detailly explained. In the end, each parent had to sign a consent form before the daughter was administered the first dose of Cervarix®.

Estimated target population

The pyramid of Cameroon's population displays an essentially young population. The statistics of the Cameroon population in 2018 read as follows:

0-14 years: 42.15% (male 5,445,142 /female 5,362,166) [37]

If Cameroon's population is 25.000.000 inhabitants, the estimated population of girls from 0-14 in Buea with a population of 200.000 inhabitants is 42.897 [37].

Furthermore, the number of girls from 9-13 years old is estimated at 1.494.239 for the whole country (39). With a population growth rate of 2,6 % per year [39], the estimated population for girls aged between 9-13 years is 11.954 and 9.975 respectively for Buea and Mutengene (40).

RESULTS

Research instrument and Data Collection
The data instrument was case report forms (CRF). The case report form contained sections to capture the demographic characteristics of participants and their parents/guardians.

Study variables
The dependent variables in this study were the general characteristics of parents/guardians and study participants. The Independent variable was the parents' age.

Statistical Analysis
Data was captured into Microsoft Excel Office 2018 (Microsoft Inc) and exported to Statistical Package for Social Scientist (SPSS) version 25.0 for statistical analysis. Categorical variables are presented as frequency tables and numerical variables as descriptive measures expressed as mean ± standard deviation (SD). The association between parents' age and demographic characteristics was assessed using bivariate and multivariate logistic regression analyses. Odds ratios (O.R) and Chi-square ($\chi2$) tests were used to compare parents' age with other characteristics and participants' characteristics. P-values ≤ 0.05 were considered significant.

RESULTS

A total of 101 girls with mean (± SD) age 12.22 ± 2.03 years were consecutively enrolled in this study. Of the 101 participants, 65 (64.4%) and 33 (32.7%) were from Buea and Mutengene respectively. 94.1 % of parents who accompanied their daughters for vaccination were female.
 their general characteristics are presented in Table 1.

Table 3: Parents' characteristics

Variable	Subclass	Parents' age groups (years)		Total (%)	χ^2	p-value
		20 – 40 (%)	> 40 (%)			
Parents						
Occupation	Skilled	48 (69.6)	29 (90.6)	77 (76.2)	5.416	0.067
	Business	5 (7.2)	1 (3.1)	6 (5.9)		
	Student	16 (23.2)	2 (6.3)	18 (17.8)		
Education	Primary	4 (5.8)	1 (3.1)	5 (5.0)	0.717	0.699
	Secondary	21 (30.4)	12 (37.5)	33 (32.7)		
	University	44 (63.8)	19 (59.4)	63 (62.4)		
Marital status	Unmarried	26 (37.7)	7 (21.9)	33 (32.7)	2.483	0.115
	Married	43 (62.3)	25 (78.1)	68 (67.3)		
Sex	Male	3 (4.3)	3 (9.4)	6 (5.9)	0.989	0.320
	Female	66 (95.7)	29 (90.6)	95 (94.1)		
	Total	*69*	*32*	*101*		

The majority, 69% of parents who brought their children for vaccination, were aged between 20 to 40 years.

Graphic representation of some characteristics of parents

Chart 1: OCCUPATION

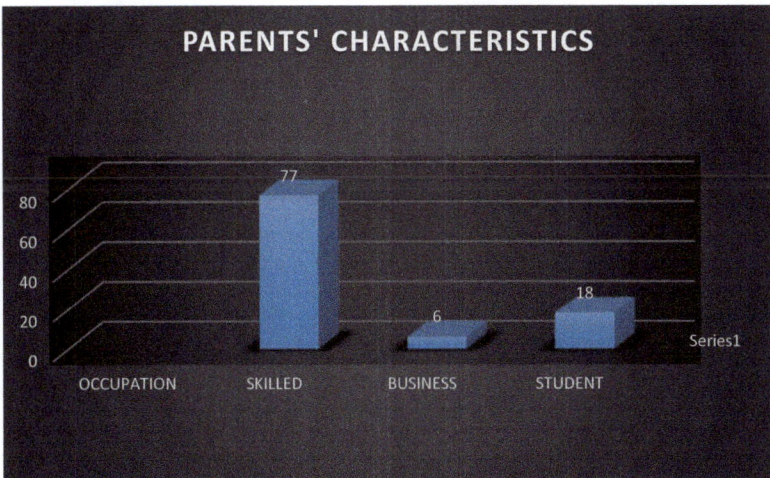

Skilled occupation towers the diagram with 76.2 % while the category business craws with a Lilliputian value of 5.9 %.

Chart 2 : EDUCATION

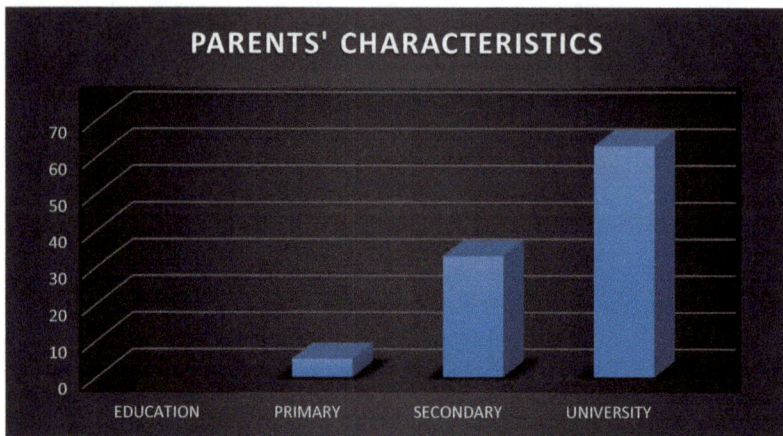

In the matter of education, cumulatively, both secondary and tertiary education represents the crushing majority of 95 % compared with the meager 5 % for primary education.

Table 2: Association of parent's age with daughters' characteristics

Parent's age groups (years)

Variable	Subclass	20 – 40 (%)	> 40 (%)	Total (%)	χ^2	*p*-value
Daughters						
Education	Primary	32 (46.4)	13 (40.6)	45 (44.6)	0.298	0.588
	Secondary	37 (53.6)	19 (59.4)	56 (55.4)		
Age groups (years)	≤ 14	56 (81.2)	24 (75.0)	80 (72.9)	0.504	0.478
	15	13 (18.8)	8 (25.0)	21 (20.8)		
Cervarix doses	Incomplete	12 (17.4)	8 (25.0)	20 (19.8)	0.797	0.372
	Complete	57 (82.6)	24 (75.0)	81 (80.2)		
	($\bar{x} \pm SD$)	12.12 ± 2.04	12.44 ± 2.03	12.22 ± 2.03	0.545	0.462
	Total	*69*	*32*	*101*		

56% of girls aged between 9 to 14 years were already in secondary school. 21 (20.8 %) incorporated in this study had just 15. 81 (80.2%) completed all the doses of vaccines required.

Table 3: Multinomial logistic regression of parents and participants characteristics in association with parent's age

Variable	Subclass	p-value	χ^2	O.R (95% C.I)
Parents				
Occupation	Skilled	$2.75 \times 10^{-3}*$	12.368	0.1 (0.0 – 0.4)
	Business	0.42		0.3 (0.0 – 5.0)
	Student	Ref		1.0
Education	Primary	0.77	7.892	1.6 (0.1 – 30.1)†
	Secondary	$1.06 \times 10^{-2}*$		0.2 (0.0 – 0.7)
	University	Ref		1.0
Marital status	Unmarried	0.17	1.985	2.1 (0.7 – 6.3)
	Married	Ref		1.0
Sex	Male	0.50	0.469	0.5 (0.1 – 4.0)
	Female	Ref		1.0
Participants				
Education	Primary	0.72	0.129	1.2 (0.5 – 2.9)†
	Secondary	Ref		1.0
Age groups (years)	≤ 14	0.49	0.469	1.4 (0.5 – 4.2)†
	15	Ref		1.0
Cervarix doses	Incomplete	0.315	0.989	0.6 (0.2 – 1.6)
	Complete	Ref		1.0

The occupation of the parents was the independent predictor for showing up for the vaccine .

Skilled occupation and secondary school educational level had statistically significant values. Girls ≤ 14 years, evidently had more odds to be incorporated in our study.

DISCUSSION

The health authorities have an uphill task to reverse the present trend. Hesitancy against Cervical cancer vaccination seems deeply rooted in society [41]. The Ministry of Public Health (MPH) and all its ramifications on the national territory have to engage in profound sensitization of the society. The community leaders, who are, the chiefs of villages and quarters should be coopted. the leaders of the mainstream religious bodies should be associated. Unorthodox "Men of God" claiming to have magical powers to cure any disease should be brought to order [42,43,44]. At every Ante-Natal Clinic (ANC), and, Infant Welfare Clinic (IWC), health personnel should be trained to deliver during Education- Instruction-Communication (EIC) activity, a talk on cervical cancer. Pediatricians should be put at contribution to educate parents on the importance of the vaccine against HPV [45,46,47]. Traditional birth attendants in villages where there are no health units should also join the cohort of educators. Short spots talking about cervical cancer should be broadcasted over national and private radio stations and televisions. Educational authorities should include in school curricula, basic notions about gynecological cancers [42].

In our study, 20 % of the participants did not complete their vaccines. Although a single shot of vaccine gives some degree of protection [48], it is advisable to have the complete doses, that is the initial dose, the second dose 2 months later, and the 3rd dose 6 months later if the participant is from 15 years upwards [48], for maximum protection. There are also cross-protection benefits against other species derived from administration of the normal doses. There is protection against Genito-anal, and oral diseases caused by HPV [49].

In our study, subclass secondary education is statistically significant. With many studies, we are in accordance that education has a pivotal role to play in the fight against cervical cancer [42]. People with little or no education have the weakness to believe in myths, folktales, and witchcraft. They drain away from health services which could have been of help to them and instead rely on unscrupulous "Men of God", herbalists, and witch doctors [42]. The higher the education, the more cartesian is one's mindset. There is an understanding of the pathology and the means of prevention and treatment. One is not overwhelmed by the "mysticism" hovering sadly around cervical cancer, ferried by the ordinary man in the society [50]. The more educated one is, the more one seeks rational solutions.

Our findings are in line with those of many authors as far as the financial capacitation of the woman is concerned. 77 % of parents who presented themselves with their daughters, had skilled occupations (doctors, lecturers, lawyers, nurses, teachers, , etc.). Men have an influence on decisions patterning to health issues [42], but financial empowerment brought along by the occupation of the woman makes her less dependent if not independent from their spouse. She can take decisions on health issues concerning the family [42,51,52,53,54,55].

94 % of parents who brought their daughters for vaccination were women. Despite their occupation, women seem more empathic, caring, and can allocate time for family health issues. They have a protective behavior towards their offsprings [56].

CONCLUSION

Admits social upheaval against vaccination the health authorities should use all available means of sensitization to create awareness between HPV infection, cervical cancer, and other HPV related anogenital diseases. Financial empowerment and level of education play a pivotal role in women bringing their daughters for vaccination against HPV.

ACKNOWLEDGMENT

We are thankful to the Cameroon- Arizona partnership (CAP) project for the supply of vaccines. Special thanks to Dr. David Greenspan, who worked hard for the donation of vaccines.

We are grateful to the Baptist Heath Services complex in Mutengene for the storage of vaccines.

RECOMMENDATIONS

On the heels of these findings, we recommend another study to try to find out some of the reasons why there is hesitancy towards cervical cancer vaccination.

REFERENCES

1. Kafuruki L, Rambau PF, Massinde A, Masalu N. Prevalence and predictors of Cervical Intraepithelial Neoplasia among HIV infected women at Bugando Medical Centre, Mwanza-Tanzania. Infect Agent Cancer. 2013;8:45.
2. Cameroon: Human Papillomavirus and Related Diseases, Summary Report 2015 - CMR.pdf. [cited 2020 Feb 10]. Available from: http://www.hpvcentre.net/statistics/reports/CMR.pdf

3. Franco EL, Duarte–Franco E, Ferenczy A. Cervical cancer: epidemiology, prevention and the role of human papillomavirus infection. CMAJ. 2001;164:1017–25.

4. Tota JE, Chevarie–Davis M, Richardson LA, Devries M, Franco EL. Epidemiology and burden of HPV infection and related diseases: implications for prevention strategies. Prev Med. 2011;53(suppl 1):S12–21. doi: 10.1016/j.ypmed.2011.08.017. [PubMed]

5. Arbyn M, Castellsague X, de Sanjose S, et al. Worldwide burden of cervical cancer in 2008. Ann Oncol. 2011;22:2675–86. doi: 10.1093/annonc/mdr015.

6. Sarah Finocchario-Kessler, Catherine Wexler et al.Cervical cancer prevention and treatment research in Africa: a systematic review from a public health perspective. *BMC Women's Health* volume 16, Article number: 29 (2016)

7. Mamsau Ngoma and Philippe Autier. Cancer prevention: cervical cancer. Ecancermedicalscience. 2019; 13: 952.Published online 2019 Jul 25. doi: 10.3332/ecancer.2019.952

8. Fidler MM, Soerjomataram I, Bray F. A global view on cancer incidence and national levels of the Human Development Index. *Int J Cancer.* 2016;139(11):2436-2446.

9. Varghese C, Carlos MC, Shin HR. Cancer burden and control in the Western Pacific region: challenges and opportunities. *Ann Glob Health.* 2014;80(5):358-369.

10. Shrestha AD, Neupane D, Vedsted P, Kallestrup P. Cervical cancer prevalence, incidence and mortality in low and middle income countries: a systematic review. *Asian Pac J Cancer Prev.* 2018;19(2):319-324.

11. Vaccarella S, Lortet-Tieulent J, Plummer M, Franceschi S, Bray F. Worldwide trends in cervical cancer incidence: impact of screening against changes in disease risk factors. *Eur J Cancer.* 2013;49(15):3262-3273.

12. Holme F, Kapambwe S, Nessa A, Basu P, Murillo R, Jeronimo J. Scaling up proven innovative cervical cancer screening strategies: challenges and opportunities in implementation at the population level in low- and lower-middle-income countries. *Int J Gynaecol Obstet.* 2017;138(suppl 1):63-68.

13. World Health Organization. *Assessing National Capacity for the Prevention and Control of Noncommunicable Diseases: Report of the 2017 Global Survey.* Geneva, Switzerland: World Health Organization; 2018. https://apps.who.int/iris/bitstream/handle/10665/276609/9789241514781-eng.pdf. Accessed December 12, 2019.

14. Institute for Health Metrics and Evaluation. *Financing Global Health 2018: Countries and Programs in Transition.* Seattle, WA: Institute for Health Metrics and

Evaluation;2019. http://www.healthdata.org/sites/default/files/files/policy_report/FGH/2019/FGH_2018_full-report.pdf. Accessed September 28, 2019.

15. Weyinshet Gossa, Michael D Fetters. How Should Cervical Cancer Prevention Be Improved in LMICs?AMA J Ethics. 2020 Feb 1;22(2):E126-134. doi: 10.1001/amajethics.2020.126.

16. Kabakama S, Gallagher KE, Howard N, et al. Social mobilisation, consent and acceptability: a review of human papillomavirus vaccination procedures in low and middle-income countries. *BMC Public Health*. 2016;16(1):834.

17. Lane S, MacDonald NE, Marti M, Dumolard L. Vaccine hesitancy around the globe: analysis of three years of WHO/UNICEF Joint Reporting Form data-2015-2017. *Vaccine*. 2018;36(26):3861-3867.

18. International Agency for Research on Cancer, World Health Organization. Cancer fact sheets: cervix uteri. http://gco.iarc.fr/today/data/factsheets/cancers/23-Cervix-uteri-fact-sheet.pdf. Published March 2019. Accessed April 10, 2019.

19. Cunningham MS, Davison C, Aronson KJ. HPV vaccine acceptability in Africa: a systematic review. Prev Med. 2014;69:274–9.

20. Hopkins TG, Wood N. Female human papillomavirus (HPV) vaccination: Global uptake and the impact of attitudes. Vaccine. 2013;31(13):1673–9.

21. Sankaranarayanan R, Budukh AM, Rajkumar R. Effective screening programmes for cervical cancer in low- and middle-income developing countries. Bull World Health Organ. 2001;79(10):954–62.

22. Gaffikin L, Blumenthal PD, Emerson M, Limpaphayom K, Royal Thai College of Obstetricians and Gynaecologists (RTCOG)/JHPIEGO Corporation Cervical Cancer Prevention Group [corrected]. Safety, acceptability, and feasibility of a single-visit approach to cervical-cancer prevention in rural Thailand: a demonstration project. Lancet Lond Engl. 2003;361(9360):814–20.

23. Blumenthal PD, Gaffikin L, Deganus S, Lewis R, Emerson M, Adadevoh S. Cervical cancer prevention: safety, acceptability, and feasibility of a single-visit approach in Accra, Ghana. Am J Obstet Gynecol. 2007;196(4):407. e1–407.e9.

24. Castro W, Gage J, Gaffikin L, Sellors J, Sherris J. Effectiveness, Safety, and Acceptability of Cryotherapy: A Systematic Literature Review. [Internet]. Seattle: Path; 2003. Available from: http://www.path.org/publications/detail.php?i=687. Accessed 6 July 2015.

25. Apgar BS, Kaufman AJ, Bettcher C, Parker-Featherstone E. Gynecologic procedures: colposcopy, treatments for cervical intraepithelial neoplasia and endometrial assessment. Am Fam Physician. 2013;87(12):836–43.

26. Muruka K, Nelly MR, Gichuhi W, Anne-Beatrice K, Eunice CJ, Rose KJ. Same day colposcopic examination and loop electrosurgical excision procedure (LEEP) presents minimal overtreatment and averts delay in treatment of cervical

intraepithelial neoplasia in Kenyatta National Hospital, Kenya. Open J Obstet Gynecol. 2013;03(03):313–8.

27. Sarah Finocchario-Kessler, Catherine Wexler, May Maloba, Natabhona Mabachi, Florence Ndikum-Moffor & Bukusi . Cervical cancer prevention and treatment research in Africa: a systematic review from a public health perspective. *BMC Women's Health* volume 16, Article number: 29 (2016)

28. Walboomers JM, Jacobs MV, Manos MM, Bosch FX, Kummer JA, Shah KV, et al. Human papillomavirus is a necessary cause of invasive cervical cancer worldwide. J Pathol. 1999;189(1):12–9.

29. Clifford GM, Smith JS, Plummer M, Muñoz N, Franceschi S. Human papillomavirus types in invasive cervical cancer worldwide: a meta-analysis. Br J Cancer. 2003;88(1):63–73.

30. Li N, Franceschi S, Howell-Jones R, Snijders PJF, Clifford GM. Human papillomavirus type distribution in 30,848 invasive cervical cancers worldwide: Variation by geographical region, histological type and year of publication. Int J Cancer. 2011;128(4):927–35.

31. World Health Organization (WHO). Comprehensive cervical cancer prevention and control: a healthier future for girls and women [Internet]. 2013. Available from: http://apps.who.int/iris/bitstream/10665/78128/3/9789241505147_eng.pdf ?ua=1. Accessed 6 July 2015.

32. de Freitas AC, Coimbra EC, Leitão Mda CG. Molecular targets of HPV oncoproteins: potential biomarkers for cervical carcinogenesis. Biochim Biophys Acta. 2014;1845(2):91–103.

33. Flepisi BT, Bouic P, Sissolak G, Rosenkranz B. Biomarkers of HIV-associated Cancer. Biomark Cancer. 2014;3:11–20.

34. World Health Organization (WHO). Human papillomavirus vaccines: WHO position paper, October 2014 [Internet]. 2014. Available from: http://www.who.int/wer/2014/wer8943.pdf?ua=1. Accessed 6 July 2015.

35. Gallagher KE, LaMontagne DS, Watson-Jones D. Status of HPV vaccine introduction and barriers to country uptake. *Vaccine*. 2018;36(32)(pt A):4761-4767.

36. Kabakama S, Gallagher KE, Howard N, et al. Social mobilisation, consent and acceptability: a review of human papillomavirus vaccination procedures in low and middle-income countries. *BMC Public Health*. 2016;16(1):834.

37. Available:http://cvuc.cm/national/index.php /en/about-uccc/the-secretariat/142-association/carte-administrative/sud- ouest/fako/404-buea [Cited 2020 Feb 16].

38. https://cbchealthservices.org/hospitals/baptist-hospital-mutengene/: *Population of girls (1,000) 9-15 years, by single year of age, Cameroon, 2010-2015 Source: UNPD 2011.*

39. https://tradingeconomics.com/cameroon/population-growth-annual-percent-wb-data.html

40. https://www.scidev.net/afrique-sub-saharienne/author.ghislaine-deudjui.html

41. C. Neh Fru, Tassang Andrew, Frederick Nchang Cho, Tassang Thierry and P. Ngum Fru. Determinants of Awareness and Knowledge on Cervical Cancer among Women in Buea- Cameroon. International Journal of Research and Reports in Gynaecology. 3(3): 1-14, 2020.

42. Pefok JD. Fake pastors denounced. In: Cameroon Postline;2018.

43. Nzie F. Poverty, fake pastors, and church businesses. In.Cameroon. Camerounlink Int; 2014.

44. WHO Safety update of HPV vaccines
https://www.who.int/vaccine_safety/committee/topics/hpv/June_2017/en (July, 2017), Accessed 2nd Feb 2020

45. T Palmer, L Wallace, KG Pollock, *et al.*Prevalence of cervical disease at age 20 after immunisation with bivalent HPV vaccine at age 12–13 in Scotland: retrospective population study.BMJ, 365 (2019), Article l1161

46. A Phillips, C Patel, A Pillsbury, J Brotherton, K MacartneySafety of human papillomavirus vaccines: an updated review.Drug Saf, 41 (2018), pp. 329-346

47. Schiller J., Lowy D. Explanations for the high potency of HPV prophylactic vaccines. *Vaccine.* 2018;36(32):4768–4773. doi: 10.1016/j.vaccine.2017.12.079.

48. Brown DR, Kjaer SK, Sigurdsson K, Iversen OE, Hernandez-Avila M, Wheeler CM, Perez G, Koutsky LA, Tay EH, Garcia P, Ault KA, Garland SM, Leodolter S, Olsson SE, Tang GW, Ferris DG, Paavonen J, Steben M, Bosch FX, Dillner J, Joura EA, Kurman RJ, Majewski S, Muñoz N, Myers ER, Villa LL, Taddeo FJ, Roberts C, Tadesse A, Bryan J, Lupinacci LC, Giacoletti KE, Sings HL, James M, Hesley TM, Barr E. The impact of quadrivalent human papillomavirus (HPV; types 6, 11, 16, and 18) L1 virus-like particle vaccine on infection and disease due to oncogenic nonvaccine HPV types in generally HPV-naive women aged 16-26 years. J Infect Dis. 2009;199:926–935.

49. C. Neh Fru, Tassang Andrew, Frederick Nchang Cho, Tassang Thierry and P. Ngum Fru. Socio-economic Determinants Influencing Cervical Cancer Screening in Buea: A Cross-Sectional Study. International Journal of TROPICAL DISEASE & Health 41(11): 14-22, 2020.

50. Wichachai S, Songserm N, Akakul T, Kuasiri C. Effects of application of social marketing theory and the health belief model in promoting cervical cancer

screening among targeted women in 31. Sisaket Province, Thailand. Asian Pac J Cancer Prev. 2016;17(7):3505-10.

51. Bebis H, Reis N, Yavan T. Effect of health education about cervical cancer and papanicolaou testing on the behavior, 32. knowledge and beliefs of Turkish women. Int J. Gynecol Cancer. 2012;22(8):1407-12.

52. Shobeiri F, Javad MT, Parsa P, Roshanaei GH. Effects of group training based on the 33. health belief model on knowledge and behavior regarding the Pap smear test in Iranian women: A quasi-experimental study. Asian Pac J Cancer Prev. 2016;17(6):2871-6.

53. Swaminathan R, Selvakumaran R, Vinodha J, Ferlay J, Sauvaget C, Esmy 34. PO, et al. Education and cancer incidence in a rural population in South India. Cancer Epidemiol. 2009;33(2):89-93.

54. Marlow LA, Wardle J, Forster AS, Waller J. Ethnic differences in human papillomavirus awareness and vaccine acceptability. J Epidemiol Community Health. 2009;63:1010–5.

55. Poudel K, Sumi N. Analyzing awareness on risk factors, barriers and prevention of cervical cancer among pairs of Nepali High School students and their mothers. Int J Environ Res Public Health. 2019;16.

CHAPTER VI

KNOWLEDGE AND RISK FACTORS OF CERVICAL CANCER AMONG WOMEN IN TOWNS OF FAKO DIVISION- CAMEROON

Tassang Andrew, Celestina Neh Fru, Mike Robert Brady,Frederick Nchang Cho, Tassang Thierry, Ngum Fru Paulette, Tangi Gracious, and Toh Renald

ABSTRACT

Cervical cancer (CC) is a worldwide disease with 85% of new cases occurring in developing countries in general and Africa south of the Sahara in particular.

The objective of this study was to find possible factors which could affect knowledge about CC and also, some CC risk factors in our community.

A community-based cross-sectional study was carried out in Buea, Mutengene, and Tiko.

Knowledge about CC is modulated by the level of education and the young age of women. Risk factors although universal seem to vary according to the geographical area and the socio-cultural environment where one lives. Some risk factors identified are; early onset of sexual intercourse, polygamous marriages, multiple sexual partners, the sexual behaviour of the male partner , Human papilloma virus (HPV) infections, sexually transmitted diseases (STDs), Human Deficiency Virus (HIV), and history of genital warts. None enhancement of lifestyle as the voluntary refusal of cervical cancer screening and CC vaccination have also be found to be risky attitudes for CC.

Key-words: Cervical cancer, knowledge, risk factors, none enhancement of lifestyle.

About 80-90 % of cervical cancers in our countries present themselves at an advanced stage [1,2] CC is a preventable disease [3,4]. The 528.000 annual cases and more than 266. 000 lethal cases could have been greatly reduced if the symptoms were known or if patients had effective preventive programs as in developed countries. Africa South of the Sahara is deeply hit by this disease[4, 5,6]. In Cameroon, the prevalence of this disease is about 13.4 % according to some studies done on the field [7]. The incriminating agent is the human papilloma virus (HPV) [8, 9,10,11], which is found in 99.7% of cases of cervical cancer [2,12,13]. This agent is sexually transmissible [12]. There exist about 100 species[14,15,16 ,17], which are not all pathogenic. Specie 16 and 18 represent 2/3 of pathological cases [14,16, 18,19]. Some identified risk factors for CC are hygienic conditions, onset of sexual activities at a very young age, multiple sexual partners, polygamy, person leaving with HIV infection, infection with HPV, low socioeconomic status, multiple deliveries, recurrent STDs [20, 21, 22, 23].

Although risk factors are universal they do vary according to geographical locations and sociocultural peculiarities[21,22,] How do some of these risk factors affect the development of CC?

HPV: is at the epicenter of CC. This virus is detected in 99.7 % from all premalignant to invasive cancer of the cervix of the uterus [12,13, 26,27,28]. It is also found in perineal, oral, pharyngeal, and esophageal lesions [29]. There are 100 species, but not all are pathological. Species 8,11,16,18,31,33,45,52, and 58 are responsible for precancerous lesions and invasive CC [30].HPV acts through the help of its oncoproteins E6 and E7. These oncoproteins have a deleterious effect on the major tumor suppressors; retinoblastoma and P53. Furthermore, they get integrated into the host cell's DNA and distort the normal functioning of the infected cells. This brings about the malfunctioning of the sense of contact, cellular control, immune response, and apoptosis[31]

HIV: women younger than 25 years generally clear the cervical HPV infection because of their strong immune system [14]. Women with HIV have higher odds of being infected with oncogenic HPV [32, 33] Immune suppression in presence of HPV will lead to permanent infection of the cervix of the uterus by the HPV, with time this could lead to the development of cervical dysplasia [34,35]. A good immune system will combat cancer cells as well as slowing down their growth and development[36]

Chlamydia trachomatis: is a sexually transmitted disease that can cause inflammation of the genital tract, leading to infertility. In general, this infection is asymptomatic [36]. Its DNA has been found in about 40 % of cervical invasive cancers [37]. The presence of chlamydia alongside the chronic inflammation leading to dysplasia makes it more difficult to clear off the HPV.[38] . this brings along a concentration of E6 and E7 oncogenes with their clinical expression.

Furthermore, the presence of antibodies directed against chlamydia carries the odds of 1.8 being associated with squamous epithelial cancer [1]. the higher the antibodies, the higher the odds in women less than 55 years old.

Smoking: Smoking is considered as one of the most important cofactors in the genesis of CC [39, 40, 41,42]. Nicotine has been detected in the cervical mucous of women having CC [36]. Women who smoke have twice the chance of developing CC. The risk is proportional to the number of cigarettes smoked [36]. The chances of developing CC are halved after 10 years in women who stopped smoking [39,40,41,42]. Nicotine and byproducts do not only alter the DNA but also induce a local immune depression in cervical squamous cells, making it possible for HPV to strive [43].

Early-onset of sexual activities: It is thought that the cervix is immature mostly below 18 years. The local immunity is wanting, so the cervix cannot defend itself. HPV can settle on such cervixes on a chronic mode [44,45,46,47,48,49]

Multiple sexual partners: HPV is a sexually transmissible disease. The risk of infection is proportionate to the number of sexual partner. [50,51,52] About 75% of women will be exposed to HPV during their sexual life [14,53]

Multiple parities: Multiple pregnancies are synonymous with repeated cervical trauma. This renders the cervix more vulnerable. Multiple sexual encounters spread over long periods could be a risk factor depending on the individual's social behavior and immune status [54,55,56]

Low economic social status: Capacitating the woman financially will go a long way towards facilitating independence in health related decisions   [57,58]. Women with a low social status fight for daily survival and will accord less attention to health issues, mostly in the domain of prevention. Even if they are aware of some health problems, they will hardly go to a hospital because of lack of money [14,57,59]. At the level of the country, the situation is not better. Screening exercises are rare because of a lack of resources and manpower. The skeletal health system looks overwhelmed. Efficient long term follow up of patients, referral and counter referral systems, traceability, cohort follow up of patients are all wanting [60, 61,62]

Level of education: Awareness and knowledge about CC rise according to the level of education. Some people with little or no education are even ignorant of the existence of CC. With a high level of education, many women are aware of symptoms of the disease and go out in search of preventive measures and rational treatment [30,57,60].

The objective of our study is to describe knowledge level and risk factors of CC in women in towns of Fako division- Cameroon.

MATERIALS AND METHODS

Study design, sample population, and strategy.

This was a community-based cross-sectional study carried out from the 5th to 20th of January 2021, in three communities; Buea, Mutengene, and Tiko in the Fako Division-Cameroon. Buea and its environment have a population of 200,000 inhabitants [63], Mutengene has a population of 32,936 [64] and Tiko has a mainly farming and trading population of 117,883 [65].

Ethical and administrative clearance

The Institutional Review Board – Faculty of Health Sciences (IRB-FHS) of the University of Buea approved the study and authorisations were obtained from the administration of Atlantic medical Foundation Hospital -Mutengene.

Sampling procedure

Women aged from 15 to 62 years were recruited for the study. Peer educators thoroughly explained the questionnaires and procedures to respondents, as well as assuring them of anonymity and confidentiality. Questionnaires were then administered to those who consented. Pregnant women and those with a history of total hysterectomy were excluded from the study.

Sample size determination

The sample size was calculated using the CDC-Epi InfoTM 7.2.3.1 StatCalc software, with the following characteristics: an estimated population size for Fako Division of 120,000 inhabitants[65], expected frequency of persons living with cervical cancer in Cameroon of 13.8 % [66], accepted error margin of 5%, design effect of 1.0 and one clusters. Thus, the CDC-Epi InfoTM 7.2.3.1 StatCalc estimated minimum sample size was 183.

Research instrument and Data Collection

The data instrument (paper-based questionnaire) was adapted from a related study[57]. The questionnaire contained sections to capture demographic characteristics, awareness, and knowledge of cervical cancer. Trained peer-educators / nurses administered the questionnaires. A pilot session of the questionnaire was done before the survey to ensure that respondents were able to understand it and that questions were interpreted as intended.

Knowledge of cervical cancer was assessed on six questions (Table 2); five of which were True/False/I don't know and one Yes/ No question. A negative response was assigned a score of '1', and a positive response '0' for the Yes/No question. All of the

True / False questions were considered true. Responses for these questions were coded as '1' for a correct ("True") and '0' for an incorrect response ("False/I don't know"). A composite score was derived for each respondent . Composite scores of 5 – 6 were considered a highly knowledge level , 3 – 4 were considered a medium level knowledge. Scores of 1-2 were considered to indicate a low knowledge level.

Study variables

The dependent variable in this study was the knowledge level score, determined as describe above. Independent variables were respondents' general characteristics.

Statistical Analysis

Data was captured into Microsoft Excel Office 2018 (Microsoft Inc) and exported to CDC-Epi InfoTM 7.2.3.1 (CDC-Epi InfoTM, USA) for statistical analysis. Categorical variables are presented as frequency tables and the association between knowledge of cervical cancer (none/low/ medium) and demographic characteristics were assessed using bivariate analysis, and multivariate logistic regression analyses. Odds ratios (O.R) and Chi-square ($\chi2$) tests were used to compare participants' characteristics with knowledge of cervical cancer. P-values ≤ 0.05 were considered significant.

Limitations and Strengths of the Study

The data that was acquired from the questionnaire completely depended on self-reported accounts of respondents. However, questionnaires were pre-tested and administered by trained peer-educators or nurses.

RESULTS

A total of 250 consecutively enrolled participants were included in this analysis; their general characteristics are presented in Table 1.

Table 1: General characteristics of study participants

Characteristic	Subclass	Frequency (%)
Age groups (Years)	15 – 20	55 (22.0)
	21 – 30	62 (24.8)
	31 – 40	60 (24.0)
	41 – 50	43 (17.2)
	> 50	30 (12.0)
Age of first sex (Years)	15 – 20	145 (58.0)
	21 – 25	68 (27.2)
	26 – 30	26 (10.4)
	31 – 35	9 (3.6)
	36 – 40	2 (0.8)
Education	No Formal Education	25 (10.0)
	Primary	52 (20.8)
	Secondary	78 (31.2)
	Tertiary	95 (38.0)
Marital status	Single	97 (38.8)
	Married	130 (52.0)
	Divorcee	5 (2.0)
	Widow	18 (7.2)
Residence	Buea	82 (32.8)
	Mutengene	85 (34.0)
	Tiko	83 (33.2)

The ages of respondents ranged from 15 – 62 years with the overall mean (x ± SD) age being 33.2 ± 12.7 years. The largest age group of study participants were   21 – 30 years old ,with 24.8%of respondents in this group. The next most populous group was the 31 – 40 years age group at 24%, and the least being the more than 50 years age group 12%. A little more than one-third 95 (38%) of the respondents had attended tertiary education, followed by 78 (31.2%) with secondary education, 52 (20.8%) with primary and then 25 (10%) with no formal education. 52% of our sample population was married, followed by 38.8 % made of single women, then 7.2 and 2%, respectively for widows and divorcees.

Knowledge and risks of cervical cancer

Of the 250 participants, only 4 (1.6%) had previously taken the HPV vaccine. Participant's knowledge of cervical cancer is presented in Table 2.

Table 2: Knowledge of cervical cancer

Question on knowledge of cervical cancer	True	False	I don't know
Infection with HPV increases risk of cervical cancer	43 (17.2)	72 (28.8)	135 (54.0)
Cervical cancer is preventable (Y/N)	74 (29.6)	143 (57.2)	33 (13.2)
Treatment for precancerous lesion can help prevent cervical cancer	113 (45.2)	36 (14.4)	101 (40.4)
Is there a test to check if someone is infected with HPV	70 (28.0)	101 (40.4)	79 (31.6)
Is there a vaccine to prevent cervical cancer	101 (40.4)	88 (35.2)	61 (24.4)
All women infected with HPV get cervical cancer	91 (36.4)	11 (4.4)	148 (59.2)
Graded knowledge of cervical cancer		**Frequency**	**%**
0		66	26.4
1		44	17.6
2		72	28.8
3		48	19.2
4		20	8.0
No measurable knowledge		66	26.4
Low knowledge level		116	46.4
Medium knowledge level		68	22.7

54 and 28.8 % making a total of 82.8 % of our sample population cannot establish the link between HPV and cervical CC. Just 29.9 % of our sample think that CC is preventable. 54.8 % do not know that treatment of precancerous lesions can prevent CC. Just 28% are aware that there is a test to detect HPV. 59.6 % do not know of the existence of any vaccine against CC. Just 36.6% of our sample study are aware that infection with HPV could lead to CC. In our sample, nobody was highly

knowledgeable in CC. The percentages were 26.4, 46.4, and 22.7 respectively for no measurable, low and medium knowledge levels Cervical Cancer Risk / Protective Factors are presented in Table 3.

Table 3: Risk of cervical cancer

Risk of cervical cancer	Subclass	Frequency	%
Prior CC screening		43/227	17.2
Duration of previous screening (years)	0 – 3	16/207	37.2
	4 – 5	10/207	23.3
	6 – 10	12/207	27.9
	> 10	05/207	11.6
Prior treatment of CC		04/244	1.6
History of genital warts		44/250	17.6
Age of first sex	15 – 20	145/250	58.0
	21 – 25	68/250	27.2
	26 – 30	26/250	10.4
	31 – 35	09/250	3.6
	36 – 40	02/250	0.8
Number of sexual partners in the last 5 years	0 – 3	196/243	80.7
	4 – 6	46/243	18.9
	7 – 10	01/243	0.4
Is your husband having other wives		03/115	2.6
Is your husband having other sexual partners		73/240	30.4
Have you had a vaccine for HPV?		04/242	1.7
Are you HIV positive		10/231	4.3
Have you had any STI in the last one year		26/227	11.5
Are you on oral contraceptives for family planning?		34/249	13.7

Just 17.2% of our studied population had had a previous CC screening, and only 37.2 of this group had screening 0-3 years ago. 1.6 % had some prior treatment for CC. 17,6 % have a history of genital warts. 58% of our sample had their 1st sexual intercourse between 15-20 years of age. About the number of sexual partners for the last 5 years, 80.7 % had 0-3 partners, 18.9 had between 4-6 sexual partners, and 0.4 % had 7-10

sexual partners. 2.6 % of our studied population come from a polygamous marriage. 30.4 % of women interrogated affirm that their husbands have extra conjugal affairs with some other women. Just 1.7 of our sample had received an HPV vaccine. 4.3 % of our sample is HIV positive. And 11.5 % of women interrogated confirm to have had at least one episode of a sexually transmitted disease for the past year. 13.7 % are using a contraceptive method.

Association between knowledge of Cervical Cancer and patients' characteristics

Age and educational status had a significant association ($p < 0.05$) with knowledge of CC (Table 4), in both bivariate analysis and multinomial regression analysis.

Table 4: Associations between respondents' characteristics and knowledge of cervical cancer

DV →		Knowledge of cervical cancer				
Variable ↓	**Subclass**	**No (%)**	**Yes (%)**	**Total (%)**	**p-value**	**O.R (95% C.I)**
Age groups (Years)	15 – 20	2 (3.0)	53 (28.8)	55 (22.0)	9.01×10^{-4}*	0.0 (0.0 – 0.3)
	21 – 30	2 (3.0)	60 (32.6)	62 (24.8)	2.45×10^{-4}*	0.0 (0.0 – 0.2)
	31 – 40	28 (42.4)	32 (17.4	60 (24.0)	0.56	1.4 (0.5 – 4.0) †
	41 – 50	24 (36.4)	19 (10.3)	43 (17.2)	0.13	2.4 (0.8 – 7.2)†
	> 50	10 (15.2)	20 (10.9)	30 (12.0)	Ref	1.0
Education	NFE	9 (13.6)	16 (8.7)	25 (10.0)	0.27	2.3 (0.5 – 10.5)†
	Primary	18 (27.3)	34 (18.5)	52 (20.8)	0.05	2.7 (1.0 – 7.3)†
	Secondary	6 (9.1)	72 (39.1)	78 (31.2)	3.99×10^{-3}*	0.2 (0.1 – 0.6)
	Tertiary	33 (50.0)	62 (33.7)	95 (38.0)	Ref	1.0
Marital status	Single	17 (25.8)	80 (43.5)	97 (38.8)	0.69	0.7 (0.1 – 3.5)
	Married	39 (59.1)	91 (49.5)	130 (52.0)	0.26	2.5 (0.5 – 11.9)†
	Divorced	4 (6.1)	1 (0.5)	5 (2.0)	0.22	5.2 (0.4 – 72.1)†
	Widowed	6 (9.1)	12 (6.5)	18 (7.2)	Ref	1.0
Residence	Buea	24 (36.4)	58 (31.5)	82 (32.8)	0.93	1.0 (0.4 – 2.4)
	Mutengene	18 (27.3)	67 (36.4)	85 (34.0)	0.57	0.8 (0.3 – 2.0)
	Tiko	24 (36.4)	59 (32.1)	83 (33.2)	Ref	1.0
	Total	*66*	*184*	*250*		

*p-values with statistical significance, NFE; No formal education

The association between the respondents' characteristics and CC, is statistically significant for the age groups 15-20 and 21-30. The odds of not being knowledgeable about CC are increased by 2.3 and 2.7 for persons with no formal education and primary level of education respectively. On the other hand, it is statistically significant for secondary school education. Tertiary education was used as the dependent characteristic. The odds of knowing CC are increased by 2.5 and 5.2 for married women and divorcees.

DISCUSSION

Risk factors

Number of sexual partners

0.4 and 18.9 % of our study population have had respectively 7-10 and 4-6 sexual partners for the past 5 years. CC is   a sexually transmissible disease, and higher the number of partners increase the risk of being infected [12,50]. 75% of sexually active women may come in contact during their active life with the HPV [12]. In this same trend, 2.6 % of our respondents have contracted a polygamous marriage and 30.4% report that their husbands have extramarital affairs with other women [20,50, 67]. The male partner can carry the HPV from an infected partner to a non-infected female partner [68].

Age at 1st sex: 58 % of our sample population had their 1st sexual intercourse between 15- 20 years. Authors are unanimous, at this tender age ≤ 18 years of age, the cervix is immature and unable to defend itself adequately against HPV, making this age group vulnerable to HPV chronic infection [44].

HIV infection : HIV infection is a risk factor for CC [30,35]. 4.3% of our sample population is HIV +. In addition to this,11.5% of this same population affirms having had at least one episode of STI for the last year. STIs are also risk factors for HPV infections [14,30].

History of HPV-related infection: genital warts were found in 17,6 % of our sample population. About 100 species of HPV do exist and species 6,11 mostly account for genital warts [14, 69].

Lifestyle enhancement: some behavioural patterns deeply anchored in our populations are regarded as "risky". In this study, just 17.2% had had a previous CC screening done. In this group, 62.8 % were screened for CC more than 3 years ago. From the onset of the premalignant lesion to cancer of the cervix, the time length could span from 10 to

15 years[29,63]. This is the reason why screening is advisable every 3 years to avoid any unpleasant surprise [29,63]. Just 1.7 % of our studied population has been effectively vaccinated. vaccination is one of the primary methods of prevention of CC, and, it has been proven to be very effective [64,65].

KNOWLEDGE

Education

Education is pivotal in the acquisition of knowledge, all researchers converge view on this [57,70,71,72]. The more a woman is literate, the sharper is her sense of judgment. Her mindset is tilted towards rational thinking. Formal education exposes one to new concepts. Knowledge could be acquired formerly and permits the learner to understand the intricacies of the disease [57]. In our study, the bulk of our sample, 72.8% was rather not at all knowledgeable or lowly knowledgeable. Just 22.7 % were averagely knowledgeable.

Age groups.

The age groups 15-20 and 21-30 are statistically significant as far as knowledge is concerned. This is owed to the demographic structure of Cameroon's population, with an essentially young population[73-74]. It is also at this age that secondary and tertiary levels of education are attained. The reason may be the youthful pattern of Cameroon's population and school

Marital status

Some sub-components in the marital status seem to be favorable for the acquisition of knowledge about CC. 2.5 and 5.2% are the increased chances in married and divorcees to be more knowledgeable in matters patterning to CC. For the former, the reason may be that they are engaged in a stable relationship so more attention is accorded to health issues. For the latter, they may be aware of the fact that they belong to a risk group, and they do their best to acquire knowledge regarding some health issues.

CONCLUSION

Although preventable, CC continues to constitute a real burden on the fragile health structures of developing countries.

First sexual intercourse at a very young age, multiple sexual partners, the male sexual factor, people living with HIV, history of genital warts and STDs, have been identified as possible risk factors for CC.

Some personal decisions as not attending CC screening and none acceptance of vaccination against HPV are regarded as deleterious for the fight against CC.

Acquisition of knowledge is a function of the level of education. The higher one is learned, the better the knowledge on CC. In this study, young age is also a contributory factor for the acquisition of knowledge.

REFERENCES

1. Zohre Momenimovahed and Hamid Salehiniya. Incidence, mortality and risk factors of cervical cancer in the world. *The Vietnamese Journal of Biomedicine* Vol 4 No12(2017) /1795-1811 Reviews.
2. Tassang Andrew et al. Cervical Cancer Screening in a Low–Resource Setting: Buea-Cameroon . International Research Journal of Oncology. 3(3): 47-55, 2020; Article no.IRJO.61096 .
3. W. A. Leyden, M. M. Manos, A. M. Geiger, S. Weinmann, J. Mouchawar, K. Bischoff, S. H. Taplin. Cervical cancer in women with comprehensive health care access: Attributable factors in the screening process. Journal of the National Cancer Institute. 2005; 97(9) : 675-683
4. Kafuruki L, Rambau PF, Massinde A, Masalu N. Prevalence and predictors of cervical intraepithelial neoplasia among HIV infected women at Bugando Medical Centre, Mwanza-Tanzania. Infect Agent Cancer. 2013;8(45).
5. Franco EL, Duarte–Franco E, Ferenczy A. Cervical cancer: Epidemiology, prevention and the role of human papillomavirus infection. CMAJ. 2001;164:1017–25.
6. Tota JE, Chevarie–Davis M, Richardson LA, Devries M, Franco EL. Epidemiology and burden of HPV infection and related diseases: Implications for prevention strategies. Prev Med. 2011;53(1):12–21. DOI: 10.1016/j.ypmed.2011.08.017. [Pub Med]
7. World Health Organization. International Agency for Research on Cancer. Cameroon Source: Globocan 2020
8. L. A. Torre, F. Islami, R. L. Siegel, E. M. Ward, A. Jemal. Global cancer in women: burden and trends. AACR. 2017
9. F. X. Bosch, N. Muñoz. The viral etiology of cervical cancer. Virus Research. 2002; 89(2) : 183-190

10. E. J. Crosbie, M. H. Einstein, S. Franceschi, H. C. Kitchener. Human papillomavirus and cervical cancer. Lancet. 2013; 382(9895) : 889-899

11. N. Heydari, M. A. Oskouee, T. Vaezi, Z. Shoja, H. A. Esmaeili, R. Hamkar, S. Jalilvand. Type-specific human papillomavirus prevalence in cervical intraepithelial neoplasia and cancer in Iran. Journal of Medical Virology. 2017

12. Sarah Finocchario-Kessler, Catherine Wexler et al. Cervical cancer prevention and treatment research in Africa: a systematic review from a public health perspective. BMC Women's Health. 2016; 16(29).

13. Clifford GM, Smith JS, Plummer M, Muñoz N, Franceschi S. Human papillomavirus types in invasive cervical cancer worldwide: A meta-analysis. Br J Cancer. 2003;88(1):63–73.

14. Tassang Andrew et al. Vaccination against Cervical Cancer: Profile of Accommodating Parents and Some Suggestions to Overcome Hesitancy against Vaccination. Journal of Cancer and Tumor International. 10(4): 33-43, 2020; Article no.JCTI.64049 ISSN: 2454-7360

15. M. A. A. Siddiqui, C. M. Perry. Human papillomavirus quadrivalent (types 6, 11, 16, 18) recombinant vaccine (Gardasil®). Drugs. 2006; 66(9) : 1263-1271

16. A. Monie, C.-F. Hung, R. Roden, T. C. Wu. CervarixTM: A vaccine for the prevention of HPV 16, 18-associated cervical cancer. Biologics. 2008; 2 : 107

17. P. Bonanni, B. Zanella, F. Santomauro, C. Lorini, A. Bechini, S. Boccalini. Safety and perception: What are the greatest enemies of HPV vaccination programmes?. Vaccine. 2017

18. International Agency for Research on Cancer, World Health Organization. Cancer fact sheets: Cervix uteri; 2019. Available:http://gco.iarc.fr/today/data/factsheets/cancers/23-Cervix-uteri-fact-sheet.pdf Published March 2019. Accessed on April 10, 2019.

19. Cunningham MS, Davison C, Aronson KJ. HPV vaccine acceptability in Africa: a systematic review. Prev Med. 2014;69:274–9.

20. Mamsau Ngoma and Philippe Autier. Cancer prevention: Cervical cancer. Ecancermedicalscience. 2019;13:952. Published online 2019 Jul 25. DOI:10.3332/ecancer.2019.952

21. S. Vaccarella, M. Laversanne, J. Ferlay, F. Bray. Cervical cancer in Africa, Latin America and the Caribbean, and Asia: Regional inequalities and changing trends. International Journal of Cancer. 2017; 141(10) : 1997-2001

22. F. X. Bosch, N. Muñoz. The viral etiology of cervical cancer. Virus Research. 2002; 89(2) : 183-190

23.

24. E. Roura, X. Castellsagué, M. Pawlita, N. Travier, T. Waterboer, N. Margall, I. T. Gram. Smoking as a major risk factor for cervical cancer and pre-cancer:

Results from the EPIC cohort. International Journal of Cancer. 2014; 135(2) : 453-466

25. S. Vaccarella, J. Lortet-Tieulent, M. Plummer, S. Franceschi, F. Bray. Worldwide trends in cervical cancer incidence: Impact of screening against changes in disease risk factors. European Journal of Cancer. 2013; 49(15) : 3262-3273

26. 60. Das BC, Gopalakrishna V, Hedau S, Katiyar S. Cancer of uterine cervix and Human Papilloma virus infection. Current Science 2000;78:52-63.

27. Walkinshaw SA, Dodgson J, McCance DJ Duncan ID. Risk factors in the development of CIN in women with vulval warts. Genitourin Med 1988;64:316-20.

28. Gallioway DA. Is vaccination against HPV a possibility? Lancet 1998;351:22-4

29. Schneider A, Koutsky LA. Natural history and epidemiological features of genital HPV infection. In: Munoz N, Bosch FX, Shah KV Meheus A, editors. The epidemiology of cervical cancer and Human Papillomavirus. Lyon: IARC; 1992. pp. 25-52.

30. Juneja A, Sehgal A,* Mitra AB,* Pandey A. A Survey on Risk Factors Associated with Cervical Cancer. Indian Cancer Society Indian Journal of Cancer, Vol. 40, No. 1, (January - March 2003)

31. E. Galani, C. Christodoulou. Human papilloma viruses and cancer in the post-vaccine era. Clinical Microbiology and Infection. 2009; 15(11) : 977-981

32. A. Ferenczy, F. Coutlée, E. Franco, C. Hankins. Human papilloma virus and HIV coinfection and the risk of neoplasias of the lower genitaltract: A review of recent developments. Canadian Medical Association Journal. 2003; 169 : 431-434 .

33. J. Palefsky. Human papillomavirus infection in HIV-infected persons. Topics in HIV medicine: a publication of the International. AIDS Society, USA. 2007; 15 : 130-133 .

34. Z. Z. Mbulawa, D. J. Marais, L. F. Johnson, A. Boulle, D. Coetzee, A.-L. Williamson. Influence of human immunodeficiency virus and CD4 count on the prevalence of human papillomavirus in heterosexual couples. The Journal of General Virology. 2010; 91(12) : 3023-3031

35. L. Pantanowitz, P. Michelow. Review of human immunodeficiency virus (HIV) and squamous lesions of the uterine cervix. Diagnostic Cytopathology. 2011; 39(1) : 65-72

36. https://www.cancer.org/cancer/cervical-cancer/causes-risks-prevention/risk-factors.html

37. P. Koskela, T. Anttila, T. Bjørge, A. Brunsvig, J. Dillner, M. Hakama, P. Lenner. Chlamydiatrachomatis infection as a risk factor for invasive cervical cancer. International Journal of Cancer. 2000; 85(1) : 35-39

38. J.S. Smith, C. Bosetti, N. Muñoz, R. Herrero, F.X. Bosch, J. Eluf-Neto, R.W. Peeling. Chlamydia trachomatis and invasive cervical cancer: Apooled analysis of the IARC multicentric case-control study. International Journal of Cancer. 2004; 111(3) : 431-439

39. J. A. Fonseca-Moutinho. Smoking and cervical cancer. ISRN Obstetrics and Gynecology. 2011; 2011

40. A. Hildesheim, R. Herrero, P. E. Castle, S. Wacholder, M. Bratti, M. Sherman, A. C. Rodríguez. HPV co-factors related to the development of cervical cancer: Results from a population-based study in Costa Rica. British Journal of Cancer. 2001; 84(9) : 1219-1226

41. J. Kim, B. K. Kim, C. H. Lee, S. S. Seo, S.-Y. Park, J.-W. Roh. Human papillomavirus genotypes and cofactors causing cervical intraepithelial neoplasia and cervical cancer in Korean women. International Journal of Gynecological Cancer. 2012; 22 : 1570-1576

42. M. Plummer, C. de Martel, J. Vignat, J. Ferlay, F. Bray, S. Franceschi. Global burden of cancers attributable to infections in 2012: A synthetic analysis. The Lancet. Global Health. 2016; 4(9) : e609-e616

43. Y. Ma, S. Collins, L. S. Young, P. G. Murray, C. B. Woodman. Smoking initiation is followed by the early acquisition of epigenetic change in cervical epithelium: A longitudinal study. British Journal of Cancer. 2011; 104(9) : 1500-1504

44. K. Louie, S. De Sanjose, M. Diaz, X. Castellsague, R. Herrero, C. Meijer, F. Bosch. Early age at first sexual intercourse and early pregnancy are risk factors for cervical cancer in developing countries. British Journal of Cancer. 2009; 100(7) : 1191-1197

45. Martin CE. Marital and coital factors in cervical cancer. Am J Pub Hlth 1967;57:803-14.

46. Rotkin ID. Epidemiology of cancer of cervix. Sexual characteristics of cervical cancer population. Am J Pub Hlth 1967;57:815-29.

47. Parazzini F, La Vecchia, Negri E, Lecchet G, Fdele L. Reproductive factors and risk of invasive and intraepithelial cervical neoplasms. Br J Cancer 1989;59:800-9.

48. Bosch FX, Munoz N, De Sanjose S, Izarzugaza I, Gili M, Viladiu P, et al. Risk factors for cervical Cancer in Columbia and Spain. Int J Cancer 1992;52:750-8.

49. Brinton LA, Famman R, Reeves WC, De Brinton RC, Gaaitan E, Tenorio F. Risk factors for cervical cancer by Histology. Gynecol Oncol 1993;51:301-6.

50. X. Castellsagué, F.X. Bosch, N. Muñoz. The male role in cervical cancer. salud pública de méxico. 2003; 45 : 345-

51. Brown S, Vessey M, Harris R. Social class, sexual habits and cancer cervix. Comm Med 1984;6:281-6.

52. Taylor RS, Carroll BE, Lloyd JW. Mortality among women in 3 catholic religious orders. Cancer 1959;12:1207-23.

53. Muruka K, Nelly MR, Gichuhi W, Anne- Beatrice K, Eunice CJ, Rose KJ. Same day colposcopic examination and loop electrosurgical excision procedure (LEEP) presents minimal overtreatment and averts delay in treatment of cervical intraepithelial neoplasia in Kenyatta National Hospital, Kenya. Open J Obstet Gynecol. 2013;03(03):313–8.

54. A. Hildesheim, R. Herrero, P. E. Castle, S. Wacholder, M. Bratti, M. Sherman, A. C. Rodríguez. HPV co-factors related to the development of cervical cancer: Results from a population-based study in Costa Rica. British Journal of Cancer. 2001; 84(9) : 1219-1226

55. J. Kim, B. K. Kim, C. H. Lee, S. S. Seo, S.-Y. Park, J.-W. Roh. Human papillomavirus genotypes and cofactors causing cervical intraepithelial neoplasia and cervical cancer in Korean women. International Journal of Gynecological Cancer. 2012; 22 : 1570-1576.

56. N. Muñoz, S. Franceschi, C. Bosetti, V. Moreno, R. Herrero, J. S. Smith, F. X. Bosch. Role of parity and human papillomavirus in cervical cancer: The IARC multicentric case-control study. Lancet. 2002; 359(9312) : 1093-1101.

57. C. Neh Fru, Tassang Andrew, F. Nchang Cho, T. Tassang and P. Ngum Fru.Socio-economic Determinants Influencing Cervical Cancer Screening in Buea: A Cross-Sectional Study. International Journal of TROPICAL DISEASE & Health. 41(11): 14-22, 2020; Article no.IJTDH.59891 ISSN: 2278–1005, NLM ID: 101632866

58. J.-Y. Kim, H.-T. Kang. Association between Socioeconomic Status and Cancer Screening in Koreans over 40 Years in Age Based on the 2010-2012 Korean National Health and Nutrition Examination Survey. Korean Journal of Family Medicine. 2016; 37(5) : 287-292.

59. Sharma HK, Prashar S. Impact of socioeconomic risk factors on carcinoma cervix: Hospital based pap smear screening of 2 years in Bihar. IP Archives of Cytology and Histopathology Research. 2018;3:39-42.

60. Neh Fru C, Tassang Andrew, Frederick Nchang Cho, Tassang Thierry and P. Ngum Fru. Determinants of awareness and knowledge on cervical cancer among women in buea- cameroon. International Journal of Research and Reports in Gynaecology. 2020;3(3):1-14.

61. Kindzeka ME. Cameroon doctors overwhelmed with patients. In. Cameroon: VOA; 2018.

62. Kaku M, Mathew A, Rajan B. Impact of socio-economic factors in delayed reporting and late-stage presentation among patients with cervix cancer in a major cancer hospital in South India. Asian Pac J Cancer Prev. 2008;9:589-94.

63. NIS. (2010). 2nd Survey on the Monitoring of Public Expenditures and the Level of Recipients' Satisfaction in the Education and Health Sectors in Cameroon (PETS₂). Retrieved from Yaoundé www.statisticscameroon.org

64. NIS. (2012). Demographic and Health survey and Multiple Indicators Cluster Survey DHS-MICS 2011. Retrieved from Yaoundé, Cameroon: www.statistics-cameroon.org

65. Fru, P. N., Cho, F N., Tassang, A. N., Fru, C. N., Fon, P. N., & Ekobo, A. S. (2021). Ownership and Utilisation of Long-Lasting Insecticidal Nets in Tiko Health District, Southwest Region, Cameroon: A CrossSectional Study. *Journal of Parasitology Research, 2021*, 1 -10. Doi:https://doi.org/10.1155/2021/8848091

66. Nkfusai, N. C., Cumber, S. N., Takang, W., Anchang-Kimbi, J. K., Yankam, B. M., Anye, C. S., . . . Anong, D. N. (2019). Cervical cancer in the Bamenda Regional Hospital, North West Region of Cameroon: a retrospective study. *Pan African Medical Journal, 32*(90). doi:10.11604/pamj.2019.32.90.18217

67. W. A. Leyden, M. M. Manos, A. M. Geiger, S. Weinmann, J. Mouchawar, K. Bischoff, S. H. Taplin. Cervical cancer in women with comprehensive health care access: Attributable factors in the screening process. Journal of the National Cancer Institute. 2005; 97(9) 675-683. International Agency for Research on Cancer, World Health Organization. Cancer fact sheets: Cervix uteri; 2019. Available:http://gco.iarc.fr/today/data/factsh   eets/cancers/23-Cervix-uteri-fact-sheet.pdf Published March 2019. Accessed on April 10, 2019.

68. Cunningham MS, Davison C, Aronson KJ. HPV vaccine acceptability in Africa: a systematic review. Prev Med. 2014;69:274–9.

69. Belglaiaa E, Souho T, Badaoui L, Segondy M, Pretet J-L, Guenat D, et al. Awareness of cervical cancer among women attending an HIV treatment center: A cross-sectional study from Morocco. BMJ Open. 2018;8:e020343

70. Thulaseedharan JV, Malila N, Hakama M, 28. Esmy PO, Cheriyan M, Swaminathan R, et al. Socio demographic and reproductive risk factors for cervical cancer – a large prospective cohort study from Rural India. Asian Pac J Cancer Prev. 2012;13(6):2991-5. 29.

71. Tadesse SK. Socio-economic and cultural vulnerabilities to cervical cancer and challenges faced by patients attending care at Tikur Anbessa Hospital: A cross sectional and qualitative study. BMC Womens Health. 2015;15(75).

72. Population of girls (1,000) 9-15 years, by single year of age, Cameroon; 2010-2015. Source: UNPD 2011.

73. Available:https://tradingeconomics.com/ca   meroon/population-growth-annual-percent- wb-data.html

www.ingramcontent.com/pod-product-compliance
Lightning Source LLC
Chambersburg PA
CBHW071137280326
41935CB00010B/1266